Flat Belly Yoga!

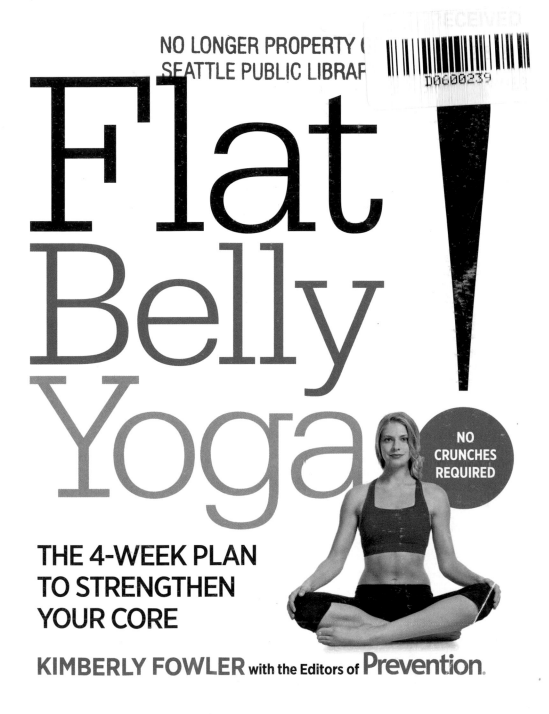

NO CRUNCHES REQUIRED

THE 4-WEEK PLAN TO STRENGTHEN YOUR CORE

KIMBERLY FOWLER with the Editors of **Prevention.**

RODALE.

Direct mail edition published by Rodale Inc. in February 2013.
Trade edition published by Rodale Inc. in August 2013.

© 2013 by Rodale Inc.

Photographs © 2013 by Rodale Inc.

Illustration by Karen Kuchar

Photographs by Beth Bischoff

Book design by Carol Angstadt

Library of Congress Cataloging-in-Publication Data is on file with the publisher.

ISBN 978–1–60961–938–1   direct hardcover
ISBN 978–1–60961–944–2   trade paperback

Distibuted to the trade by Macmillan.

2   4   6   8   10   9   7   5   3   1   direct hardcover
2   4   6   8   10   9   7   5   3   1   trade paperback

We inspire and enable people to imrove their lives and the world around them.
For more of our products visit **prevention.com**.

To those who want to
turn the dream of a Flat Belly
into a reality—
no crunches required

contents

preface

Welcome to *Flat Belly Yoga!* I'm excited that you've picked up this book—it sends a loud and clear signal that you are ready to take action. You want to feel better about your body and your health. You want the support and direction to take on what, for many of us, is a top-level challenge: tightening up our bellies. You want a program that will leave you stronger, fitter, and—let's get right down to it— looking better.

I'm excited to be going on this journey with you. I'm here to guide you as you make the transition from the couch to the yoga mat. Think of me as your personal coach as we head down this road of shedding unhealthy belly fat and gaining better, healthier lives. (We'll also have some fun along the way!)

Flat Belly Yoga! is the newest installment in the Flat Belly Diet! series and was designed with many of the same principles. So you can easily do this new, cutting-edge workout and follow the Flat Belly Diet! at the same time. The Flat Belly Diet! is effective because it not only provides a realistic path to health, but also because it *inspires* us to take that path—to change the way we think about food, about eating, and about ourselves. When you get down to it, that kind of inspiration is what enables us to change our lives.

Giving people that moment of inspiration that creates change is one of the most important things in my life. Making workouts something people feel comfortable doing (and actually look forward to) has been my primary goal since I opened my first YAS (Yoga and Spinning®) Fitness Center back in 2001.

I know how challenging it can be to set a goal and see it through. The road to *Flat Belly Yoga!*, as well as the rest of my career, has taken many twists and turns. I've faced many challenges to get here. And that's why I want to guide you through this one.

Back when I opened the original YAS Fitness Center in a rough part of Venice, California, it was a neighborhood where gunshots and police helicopters were all too frequently part of the background noise outside my studio. (Not exactly the best place for an upscale, innovative gym, right?) But I hung in there.

As my yoga workouts became more popular, the neighborhood changed around me. Today, more than 500 students come through YAS Venice each day. And the street where all this happens, Abbot Kinney Boulevard, was named "the Coolest Block in America" by *GQ* magazine in their April 2012 issue. YAS Fitness Centers has now expanded beyond YAS Venice and is headed nationwide.

One of the most gratifying aspects of this success has been being able to give back by helping people get into better shape—without a single *om*. Just to be clear, I have great respect for yoga traditions and their spiritual components. However, my goal is to transform the way everyday people—those who are simply looking for a good workout—think about yoga.

I do that by developing approachable, "no-crunch" results-oriented workouts that use the best of what yoga has to offer. The centerpiece of every one of my efforts to get people off the couch and onto the mat is an innovation in mixing the most effective parts of different exercises together. As a result, I've earned the nickname "Godmother of Hybrids." And I'll take it!

When I first opened the doors of YAS Venice, no one had ever combined yoga with indoor cycling before. And certainly, no one had dared to build a studio dedicated to the combination.

My initial hybrid workout combined hard-charging Spinning® with straightforward yoga in the same class (or in back-to-back classes). But that is just one example of a hybrid workout. Another example is my yoga-with-weights workout. Of course, these days people have come up with all kinds of hybrids: yoga and Pilates, yoga and stand-up paddle surfing, disco yoga—the combinations are endless.

Hybrid workouts have become today's most popular approach to fitness, and for good reason. The strengthening, flexibility, stress-reducing, and fat-burning benefits of modified yoga workouts combined with resistance training and/or cardio are, in so many ways, just what the doctor ordered. Good hybrid workouts provide a safe, well-rounded, and effective approach to fitness. And the Flat Belly Yoga! does this so well that you might say it is hybrid to its core (no pun intended). Combining the yoga-with-weights workouts with cardio exercise gives you a perfect storm of fat burning and core strengthening to leave your belly flatter and sassier than ever!

The whole workout plan is 32 days, which studies show is just enough time to make a lifestyle change. After your 32 days are finished, you will have the tools to keep your belly flat for life. So make sure you start with the 4-Day Jump Start, then move right into the 4-Week Workout.

To keep you inspired throughout the 32 days, I have included success stories from people just like you in every chapter. I've also included Mat Motivation sections throughout the book so that you can get to know me a little better as your coach. The Mat Motivations will also provide you with inspiration to continue moving forward as you progress in your workouts.

So whether you've put on some unwanted pounds recently or have struggled with excess weight for years, *Flat Belly Yoga!* can and will change your life. Turn the page to get started.

acknowle

dgments

Thank you to *Prevention*, Rodale, and the Rodale family for believing in me. Even when I thought I had too much on my plate with running my company, YAS Fitness Centers, you convinced me I was the right person to author *Flat Belly Yoga!* And I'm so glad you did!

I have to admit that my editor, Lora Sickora, was a dream to work with. We were definitely in sync with not only our beliefs in this project, but also our dedication to this book and the lives of its future readers. I'd also like to thank the art director, Carol Angstadt, for designing a beautiful book that embodies the Flat Belly brand.

To the test panelists who spent their summer proving that the Flat Belly Yoga! 4-Week Plan works—I so enjoyed being part of your lives and seeing you and your bellies transform. I loved watching you not only lose weight, but also gain more energy and become a lot happier than when you first began the program.

Finally, I'd like to thank my life partner, Sherri Rosen: Without you, this book would not have been finished. Your help has been invaluable—from your organizational skills (putting together a test panel was not easy), to your hidden photography talent (taking the test panelists' before and after photos), to, most of all, picking up the slack at work so I could create *Flat Belly Yoga!*

intro

duction

A Moving Experience

Gut Check

You've been sitting around for too long and it's time for a change. You're tired of trying to hide your belly under layers of clothing while secretly wishing you could still fit into those skinny jeans from 20 years ago.

I'm going to assume that if you've picked up a book called *Flat Belly Yoga!* you're hoping that exercise will help make your wish come true. Well, guess what? It can! And I'm here to guide you through the steps that can convert your fantasy into reality.

You've probably heard a thing or two about the hazards of belly fat—after all, you can hardly open up a magazine or an e-mail without seeing something about it. But what exactly is belly fat? There are actually several different types, including subcutaneous fat and visceral fat. Subcutaneous fat is basically "the inch you can pinch"—the fat you can see. Some people call it their muffin top. Excessive amounts of subcutaneous fat tell us that we are overweight or even obese.

But when you hear about dangerous belly fat, this isn't the fat people are talking about. Instead, it's visceral fat—the type of fat that hangs out in and around your internal organs. So it's hidden belly fat, and it also qualifies as the unhealthiest type of fat in your body. It has a harmful effect on your vital organs and is a major contributor to many serious health conditions, ranging from heart disease and strokes to diabetes to certain kinds of cancer.

Excess accumulation of belly fat is more dangerous than excess fat around your hips and thighs. Your genes can contribute to your being overweight and help determine where you carry this extra fat, but poor lifestyle choices can aggravate the problem. People who lead sedentary lives, for example, have more visceral fat than those who are moderately active.

In *Flat Belly Diet!* you are given the science behind losing belly fat by eating foods containing monounsaturated fatty acids, or MUFAs. These are good fats, which studies have shown may help you target that dangerous visceral fat. Similarly, *Flat Belly Yoga!* zeroes in on your muffin top with easy, fast, and portable exercise routines based on the latest research—no crunches required! And the good news is that although visceral fat is the easiest fat to put on, it's also the easiest to take off.

I'll be giving you more information on the downside of belly fat later in the book. But for now, even if your interest in *Flat Belly Yoga!* stems primarily from vanity, that's as good a starting point for success as any. And whatever your reason may be, a flatter belly is within reach. With this workout plan, you will burn belly fat in addition to other undesirable fat. You will also add muscle mass, which comes with the additional bonus of prompting your body to burn even more calories, thus moving you toward your ultimate goal of shedding even more fat!

Helping you lose unhealthy belly fat is certainly the primary goal of *Flat Belly Yoga!*, but strengthening the back and abdominal (or core) muscles surrounding your belly is a very close second. Developing a strong core yields crucial health benefits, like avoiding painful injuries to your back, neck, and hips, that cannot be achieved through dieting alone.

And on top of the health benefits, developing a strong core also directly contributes to a flatter belly—even independent of the fat you'll be burning. The transverse abdominis, just one of the major core muscles we will be making stronger through the Flat Belly Yoga! Workout acts as a muscular girdle for your stomach (think Spanx). So strengthening this muscle will automatically give your belly a flatter appearance—and it will help those skinny jeans slip on easier, too!

The Flat Belly Yoga! Workout was created as a stand-alone exercise plan, designed to free you of belly fat and strengthen your core with workouts designed and tested to help you achieve the flat belly of your dreams. But the workout is also an excellent companion to the Flat Belly Diet!, and I encourage you to use the diet and workout together. After all, research has shown that those who combine diet and exercise are more likely to lose weight and keep it off than people who only diet or only exercise. And I want you to not only achieve the flat belly of your dreams but keep it as well.

Getting Started

It's important to keep in mind that we all start at different levels. You may be a couch potato, or you may already be fairly active but still bothered by your belly fat. You may have already done yoga or some weight training in the past, or maybe you're an avid walker. Regardless of where you are beginning, we share the common goal of using the Flat Belly Yoga! Workout to combat our belly fat and strive toward a flatter stomach.

Here are five tips to help you get moving:

1. **Decide that you're going to start working out.** Only you have the power to truly commit to working out. Most of us do not have the luxury of a personal trainer who arrives at our home to get us out of bed. Assuming that this is true, the first thing you need to do is focus on and internalize your commitment to establishing a workout routine. Once you've made the decision to move forward, *Flat Belly Yoga!* moves in with a step-by-step guide to help you achieve your goal.

2. **Identify the specific motivation behind your goal.** Since you picked up a book called *Flat Belly Yoga!*, I would imagine that having a flat belly is your primary motivation, right? Losing weight or fitting into those skinny jeans could be others. Or maybe you have a class reunion or a wedding coming up. Focus on the motivation behind your goal and remind yourself of this motivation every day. It will inspire you to stick with your new workout routine, even on days when you're too busy or tired.

     Some tips that have worked for me include putting my goals on the wall in front of my computer or placing a copy of my goals by my bed so that I see them right before I go to sleep at night and when I first get up in the morning.

3. **Buy the simplest and most cost-effective equipment.** At the top of the list are a pair of walking shoes and 3-pound weights. You don't need a mat, as you can do Flat Belly Yoga! on a rug or just on the floor. But if you see a mat that you like, you might want to make the small investment. Mats are inexpensive, and you can pick one up at a sporting goods store for about $9.

     You'll also be getting in some cardio every day, so you'll need a good pair of sneakers. But don't worry—I'll provide you with more guidance on buying the right shoes in Chapter 5 on page 65.

4. **Decide when you are going to work out and *write it down*.** Finding the time to work out is always a big issue at the outset. What I've found that helps me the most is to schedule my workouts as if they are very important meetings. Also, if you're stuck on this step, you may want to check out Chapter 8 (see page 163) for some suggestions for creating time for yourself. Once you decide when the best time is for you to work out, write it down in your Flat Belly Yoga! Journal (see Chapter 9, on page 177). As you continue reading, you'll discover how keeping a journal about your exercise journey really does help you stay on track. Just remember: The more specific and thought-out your plan is, the more likely you will be to execute it.

5. **Spread the word.** Tell your friends and family what you are doing in order to increase your commitment. I know it can be a little intimidating to say,

"Hey, sis, I'm going to get a flat belly in 32 days." But choosing the wording that makes you comfortable and communicating your plan to your family and friends will make you much more firmly committed.

Take the *WORK* Out of Workout

Just as the *Flat Belly Diet!* can change the way you think about eating, *Flat Belly Yoga!* will change the way you think about working out. Together, we will take the *work* out of workout. We will adjust your mindset in order to stop thinking of working out as a painful experience akin to going to the dentist. We will transform your perception of exercise from something you're *supposed* to do into an activity you truly look forward to doing. In other words, I want your workout to be the high point of your day.

While it may seem ridiculous to think of working out in that way, I'm offering you the honest truth. Working out is the high point of my day—and by the end of the program, I'm confident it will be yours, too. But if I initially have to trick you into working out, I'm willing to do so until you have arrived at that place on your own. I know from years of my own experience, and that of countless others, that working out can and should be fun and energizing, even a release. And I know that once you get going with the right workout— the Flat Belly Yoga! Workout—you will not only see it my way, but you, too, will crave working out.

As any exercise junkie will tell you, working out is not only great for you physically but mentally as well. Nothing works better to relieve life's inevitable daily stressors than working out. Many even swear that working up a good sweat is more effective than going to a therapist. (It's certainly a whole lot cheaper!)

The benefits of working out will change your life. You will feel better about how you look. You will feel better about your health. Think about how it would feel to be able to do pretty much anything physical that may currently be out of reach—like playing sports or picking up your kids (or grandkids)—more easily and more safely.

Workouts are a great break in your day, even if they actually start it out or end it. For one thing, they get you away from work. They flood you with endorphins, those feel-good brain chemicals. They can get you out in the world or give you a break from it. They let you stop and smell the roses (why wouldn't you, you'll already be breathing better!). They can keep you connected with friends, or give you a much-needed break from people you're otherwise around all day (or all night). Workouts are *good* for you, unlike some of the other activities you may use to unwind. (Yes, recent research has shown drinking alcohol in moderation can be good for women, too—but it's hardly a healthy pastime! And watch those calories while you're at it.)

Working out is energizing, plus it gives you a chance to not be at your computer. Or sitting in traffic. Or doing laundry.

A HEALTHY CRAVING

Once you create the habit of working out, your body will begin to crave this feeling every day. You're establishing a healthy cycle that begins with you working out and concludes with you feeling better, leading you to repeat the same pattern the next day.

I know it's initially hard to find the energy to work out, but if you persist you will notice that exercising actually gives you more energy. When you don't exercise, however, your energy drops and your waist enlarges. Instead of the energizing cycle described above, you are actually perpetuating a downward cycle that is hard to break.

KEEP IT POSITIVE

Another strategy that I utilize to encourage myself is called positive self-talk (which you will learn to utilize fully in Chapter 4; see page 39). When you recognize that your internal negative voice is repeating the words *I hate working out*, you will redirect yourself toward your own positive goal by saying instead, *I would rather exercise than sit around at night.*

As you notice yourself thinking something negative in your mind, you can stop your thought midstream by saying to yourself: *Stop*. Saying this aloud will be more powerful than merely thinking it and will make you more aware of how many times you are stopping negative thoughts.

Flat Belly Yoga! Workout— The Best of All Practices

Flat Belly Yoga! combines the best of all exercise practices—strength, flexibility, and cardio—in quick and easy workouts. The number one component of *Flat Belly Yoga!* is yoga, yet it's important to remember that yoga alone will not make your stomach flat. Cardio augments the practice of yoga to burn calories and adding weights to your yoga routine serves to build muscle. There are certain carefully selected poses that we will do in the Flat Belly Yoga! Workout to strengthen your core muscles while simultaneously adding tone and definition to your abs to help flatten your stomach. In fact, the effect yoga has on your belly is two-fold: It both stretches (or elongates) and strengthens your core. Yoga requires you to create a stable platform to move in and out of poses. Doing a yoga pose correctly—and slowly!—takes a lot more core strength than doing it fast and sloppy. That's why I'm going to walk you through every pose, step-by-step. Using yoga to stretch and strengthen the core muscles during your Flat Belly Yoga! program *will* flatten your belly.

We'll keep it simple for the first 4 days with the Jump Start, which includes Yoga for Your Core (yoga without weights). Then we'll move forward step-by-step until you're ready for more challenges with Core+ Yoga, which incorporates weights into your yoga routine. I'll help you identify the level of walking that's fun, appropriate for you, and most efficient at fat burning. And whether you haven't been working out or have struggled to stick with a routine in the past, I'll share all the tricks I know to help you succeed this time around.

WORKOUT BASICS

The 4-Week Workout is divided into two categories: Core+ Yoga, composed of strength and flexibility training, and fat-blasting Heart Walk cardio sessions. Together they make the perfect combination to help you achieve the flatter, stronger belly you want. By moving at your own pace with simple-to-do exercises, you will find that you truly can take the work out of the workout.

Core+ Yoga

Core+ Yoga sessions are hybrid workouts featuring modified yoga with weights. I designed the sessions to build strength and flexibility by combining resistance training with straightforward yoga poses. Don't worry if you've never done yoga before—the yoga we do in the Core+ Yoga routines has been modified to be accessible, easy to follow, and perfect for keeping you flexible and toned.

Adding weights and resistance training to the Core+ Yoga sessions helps you build muscle mass so your body burns fat more efficiently. Don't worry about bulking up. You're won't be doing the kind of weight lifting that would bulk you up. And besides, it's basically impossible for women to muscle up like men. It takes testosterone to make those muscle bound–type bodies, and women just don't have enough of it.

What will happen is you'll develop and maintain longer, leaner, and stronger muscles while improving flexibility. In fact, yoga is the glue between weight training and cardio. You can do one or the other, but doing all three is what will make your belly fat go away.

Numerous studies have shown that lack of exercise can lead to muscle decline as we get older, starting at age 40. Combining weight training with yoga is the best way to maintain your muscle mass and strength. If you're a couch potato, by the time you're 70 years old you could lose as much as 30 percent of your lean muscle mass, and a lot of that muscle will be replaced with fat. Core+ Yoga build sstrength and muscle awareness, and if you already exercise, it will bump up your existing workout.

Heart Walk

Cardio (cardiovascular exercise) is the key to burning fat in the Flat Belly Yoga! Workout. Doing the Heart Walk cardio sessions is essential to helping you attain the flat belly you want.

The Flat Belly Yoga! Workout provides clear instructions on gauging your exertion level, so you can understand when you are in fat-burning territory. The number of calories you burn will change from week to week, calling on you to gradually increase the intensity of your cardio sessions as you advance through your 4-Week Workout Plan through interval training.

By including interval training in the Heart Walk sessions—switching between higher and lower intensities and heart rates—and by performing exercises that raise your heart rate in the Core+ Yoga series, the workout will help you maximize your fat-burning potential. In both cases, your body will burn fat more efficiently than if you simply maintain a steady heart rate. Training that raises and lowers your heart rate tricks your body into burning more calories during and after your workout as it seeks to return to its normal state.

A MOVING LIFE

More than anything, I want you to have a moving life, in every sense of the word. *Flat Belly Yoga!* was created to help you get moving and keep moving, as you say goodbye to the flabby belly of your past and hello to the flat belly awaiting you. So let's get moving!

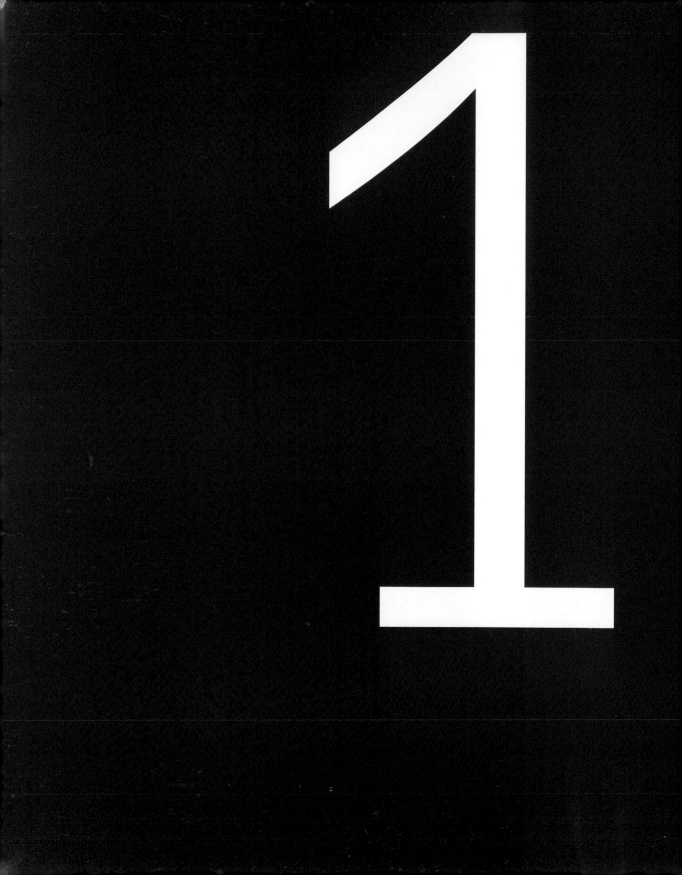

YOGA MOTION: What's in Store for Your Core?

Yoga has been around for more than 5,000 years. When it first came to the United States more than a hundred years ago, you would be more likely to experience it in a lecture hall with a professor introducing a visiting swami than actually doing yoga in a gym.

In the 1960s, yoga was thought of as one of many alternative workouts that were popular with hippies. But in the 1980s, it started to make its way into the exercise mainstream, although it still had a long way to go. Today, yoga has shed its reputation as a "woo-woo" workout. It is now firmly entrenched in the workout mainstream—more than 15 million Americans currently practice yoga in one form or another. In fact, these days you can hardly pick up a magazine or watch a television show on health or fitness that does not include yoga.

A number of scientific studies have also proven that practicing yoga is good for your overall health. It's most commonly known for decreasing stress and helping lift your mood. Most people who have never done it think of yoga as "just stretching"—and it is great for increasing flexibility. But it is much more than that. It is a whole-body workout that also improves balance and strength—especially core strength. And that's why yoga is at the core of this exercise program.

Researchers from the University of Wisconsin's Human Performance Laboratory recruited 34 healthy women for a study on the benefits of yoga. They found that regular practice of yoga significantly improved the subjects' flexibility, muscular strength, and balance. And after 8 weeks, the subjects' abdominal strength and endurance had increased significantly. The key to increasing abdominal strength was maintaining good posture while in the different yoga poses.[1]

Yoga is also great for fighting depression, anxiety, and insomnia. Studies have shown that regular yoga practice can reduce the impact of exaggerated stress responses. In this respect, yoga functions like other self-soothing techniques, such as meditation, relaxation, exercise, or even socializing with friends.[2]

You may have seen or heard reports warning that yoga can cause injuries. That is true of almost any exercise, and yoga is no exception—especially if you move too fast into the wrong kinds of poses, or repeat them too much. That is why I designed the 4-Day Jump Start—to introduce you to yoga gradually with Yoga for Your Core and reduce your risk of injury. Once you've mastered the yoga moves, you'll progress to the Core+ Yoga routine, which includes the use of weights. The yoga moves are structured around weights and increasing repetition, instead of pushing yourself further into pretzel poses. I've included Play It Safe tips throughout the book to show you how to avoid injury.

Breathe In, Breathe Out

One of the reasons you feel so good after doing yoga is because you are concentrating on your breath. Deep breathing can relax you and calm you down, which helps explain why yoga is good for stress relief. The way you breathe affects your state of mind, because your brain needs more oxygen than other parts of your body. And because we breathe in and out more than 20,000 times a day, better breathing techniques maximize your overall well-being. Poor posture or lack of body awareness may lead us to use the wrong muscles when we breathe, which results in shallow breathing.

Studies show that yoga breathing, also called *pranayama* in Sanskrit (the Indo-Aryan language of Hinduism often used in yoga instruction), can help prevent and even reverse some symptoms of diseases like chronic obstructive pulmonary disease or other stress-related illnesses. Deep-breathing exercises can also help improve lung capacity and decrease muscle tension.

When you are doing your Flat Belly Yoga! Workout, make sure you inhale through your nose and exhale through your mouth. Throughout the workout, I'll remind you when to inhale and when to exhale. So make sure you focus on your breathing—the worst thing you can do is to hold your breath, which we often subconsciously do when we're working out. Using your breath will help keep you focused on your body and the Core+ Yoga moves you are doing.

Down to the Core

These days, everyone talks about core strength—and for good reason. A strong core is crucial to getting the flat belly you want and for your overall physical conditioning. That's why Core+ Yoga is such a crucial part of the Flat Belly Yoga! Workout and lasts for 4 weeks. It's designed to work and tone your core muscles.

But what exactly is the core? When it comes to the anatomy of the core muscles, most people think the core consists only of the abdominal muscles, i.e., "abs." That's just not the case. The core is a lot more than your abs. In fact, your core muscles run from your shoulders to your hips and make up your entire torso.

Many of your core muscles can't be seen because they are buried underneath larger muscles. These hidden muscles are called *intrinsic muscles*. So it's not just about the "showy" muscles on top, called *extrinsic muscles* like the six pack.

Here are a few of the muscles we will be focusing on in your Core+ Yoga workout.

External obliques: These are the muscles just under the skin on your sides. They start on the back of the lower ribs and run on a diagonal down toward the pelvis.

Internal obliques: These muscles are underneath the external obliques. They start on the pelvis and run up toward the ribs in a diagonal line.

Transversus abdominis: This is the deepest of the four anterior abdominal wall muscles, and its job is to stabilize the lower back.

Rectus abdominis: This is the muscle responsible for the elusive six-pack. *Rectus* means straight and *abdominus* refers to the abdomen. This muscle goes straight down the abdomen.

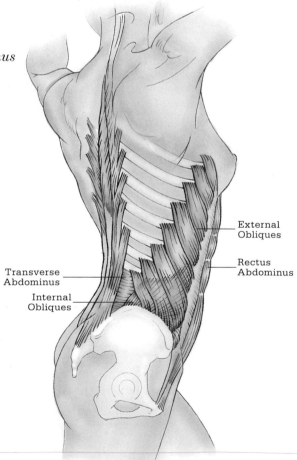

External Obliques

Rectus Abdominus

Transverse Abdominus

Internal Obliques

All of these muscles work together to keep your torso stable while your arms and legs are moving. So if your core muscles are weak, your body doesn't work as effectively and other muscles have to compensate for them. This can result in injuries such as a twisted knee, a pulled shoulder, or a bad back.

The core could be called your "center of power" because all motion and action begins with your core, especially when you exercise. The main responsibility of your core muscles is to provide enough strength to your body so it can cope with the challenges of everyday physical activity, like sitting for long periods of time. For this reason, many health and fitness experts have realized that it is more important to strengthen the core muscles than any other muscles in the body. Having a stronger core can prevent a lot of health problems.

And remember how we're going to be focusing on your breathing technique? A strong core even helps you breathe better, which improves your oxygen supply. Your core muscles participate in your exhales, helping to force air out of your lungs by squeezing your torso.

CAN YOGA MAKE YOU TALLER?

I am asked this question often, especially whenever someone starts practicing yoga. Since yoga focuses on your core and the core is responsible for your posture, the answer is yes! Your core muscles keep your back straight and your shoulders square, so they keep you from slouching. This will automatically make you look taller and make your belly look flatter.

A strong core supports good posture and proper joint alignment. Good posture not only makes you look and feel better but also prevents back pain. Good posture places the least amount of stress on your joints. A strong core keeps your neck, shoulders, hips, and knees properly aligned, which minimizes wear and tear on your body.

It also improves your back strength throughout the day. Why? Because muscles in the core are actually the ones that stabilize your whole upper and lower torso. So keeping these muscles strong will also help support proper alignment. (We'll discuss the importance of alignment more in Chapter 5.)

As you incorporate weights in your Core+ Yoga workout, we will be using yoga poses that focus on your abdominal muscles, which will strengthen your

When you build your core, you are actually preventing future problems or injuries. Here are some of the common injuries that core strength can help you avoid:

- **Lower back injuries:** This is not exactly an injury of the core, but can occur because your core is weak (the leading cause of back problems).

- **Abdominal muscle strain:** Also called a pulled abdominal muscle, this is an injury to one of the muscles of the abdominals. Normally a muscle strain occurs when the muscle is stretched too far. You'll see this with some athletes like basketball players.

- **Hernia:** A hernia is an opening or weakness in the abdominals. This causes a bulging of the abdominal wall, which is usually noticeable when the abdominal muscles are tightened and increases the pressure in the abdomen.

lower back without causing additional back strain. If your core muscles aren't strong, you can't sit up straight for long periods of time. Without a strong core, you are also more susceptible to having back problems.[3]

EXPLORE THE CORE

The Flat Belly Yoga! Workout uses specific poses to tone your core muscles. Further on in the book, I'll take you through every single pose step-by-step so that you can make the most of every movement. Chapters 6 and 7 have detailed day-by-day workouts with images to help you make sure you're holding your poses just right.

But for now, I'm going to give you a sense of how the different elements of yoga work together to give you a flat belly by presenting you with the poses featured in your workouts. We're also going to discuss why each pose has been specifically chosen for this program. So don't use this as your workout—that's coming later on. Instead, think of this as a preview of coming attractions.

Warm-Up/Breath Work

Even if you've never exercised before in your life, you probably know the importance of warming up. Every exercise program stresses the importance of not going from zero to 60—you're not a cheetah and you're not a sports car. Your body needs a little more care than that.

One theme I'm going to come back to throughout *Flat Belly Yoga!* is the importance of focusing on your breath. The beginning of every yoga practice is for paying attention to your breathing. Our bodies don't ever let us stop breathing entirely, but focusing on the breath adds a new dimension and puts us in touch with what's happening as we go from sitting to moving—or, in our lives as a whole, from sedentary to active.

Easy Spinal Twist

Warming up your lower back is also a critical part of a healthy exercise program. Your lower back, like everything from your shoulders to your hips, is part of your core. And if you don't warm up first, you can hurt yourself—that's true anywhere, but it's especially true of your lower back. (This gets truer as you age.) I don't want you to throw your back out! That would be defeating the purpose of starting an exercise program. You need to work up to it—or any workout you may do.

I find that twists can be incredibly relaxing. They take advantage of your own strength to give you a little massage without using your hands (or anyone else's). If my back gets tight, sometimes I'll drop to the floor no matter where I am (within reason) and treat myself to a spinal twist.

Rock Up to Standing

The Rock Up to Standing pose is still part of the warm-up sequence, but it takes a lot of core strength to do. I know just standing up from a seated position can be challenging at times. And the addition of weights only increases the difficulty. This can be hard the first few times you try it, and you might have to use your hands to help you stand up. But once you go from doing this pose without the weights in Yoga for Your Core to adding weights for Core+ Yoga, it will become easier.

Chair Pose

The Chair pose uses virtually every single muscle in your body. I like to use it up front in the sequence because it's an easy pose that will warm up your whole body. It takes a lot of core strength to hold yourself up in Chair pose, and the more correctly you do it, the harder it is. Now adding weights? That's a whole other ball game—one you'll be ready for by the time you progress to the 4-Week Workout.

Warrior 1 and Warrior 2

The Warrior poses are your power poses. They help you build strength and flexibility. As you concentrate on the many elements of these poses, you will start to seriously warm up your body and begin to sweat. When you start to add weights to your Warrior poses in your Core+ Yoga workout, you will be amazed at how many muscles you are using.

Plank

Plank is also in the power pose category along with Warrior 1 and Warrior 2. I don't have any push-ups in this sequence, but Plank is where a push-up starts, and you can experience a lot of the benefit of a push-up just by hanging out in plank for a little longer in each workout. You'll originally feel it in your arms, but Plank pose is 80 percent core strength, so you'll also feel it in your core. Hold it for as long as you can.

Hero Pose with a Lift

Hero pose is a core-strength pose, and since you're seated on your knees on the floor, it's a great staging ground for a little weight work. If you're doing it correctly, you will definitely break a sweat. Hero Pose with a Lift flattens your belly because it requires core strength to lift and lower your weights. To give you a visual: It looks like you are doing the wave at a baseball game.

Seated Tree—Up and Over

This is a great side stretch that works your core. It also really gives your lower body a flexibility workout. By sitting on the floor to do your core work, which is when you lift up and over, Seated Tree works your obliques. In the studio, my students call this pose "the muffin top killer."

Bridge with a Lift

Bridge is a backbend. It's one of the most common poses you'll see in advertisements or illustrations of yoga practice. I'm sure when you see the photo you'll recognize it! Bridge really works the front of your body, giving you a great stretch that activates your core. And while it works your front, it also strengthens your lower back. Everything from your hips to your torso is included in your core, and Bridge gets it all.

Corpse

In the Corpse pose, you're simply lying on the floor. You're breathing and relaxing—and that's it. (I know you may be thinking, "I'm already an expert at this one.") While it sounds like nap time from kindergarten, a few minutes in Corpse pose happens to be one of the most important parts of a yoga workout.

One of the things that inspired me to take my yoga classes at my studio down to a 1-hour duration was the fact that my busy students had been leaving before they got to their relaxation pose. If you cut out breath work and relaxation, then you're really just doing a little stretching. You're not really doing yoga. The Corpse pose at the end gives you a couple of minutes to have your body adjust to the workout you just did.

Have you ever gone for a massage, then realized at the end of it you were late for your next appointment? So you rolled right off that massage table and got right into traffic, and guess what? You wasted your massage. Your body became tense again. It's the same with wrapping up your yoga practice with a Corpse pose. By really making sure you get a transitional phase in between sweating and stretching and going back to your day, you are protecting your investment in your exercise program.

Upright Rows

"Sit up straight" isn't just a command from your mother—it's the key to doing this pose correctly. And this pose is one hard stretch. You're going to want to roll forward, but it takes a lot of effort to sit up straight and do it correctly. An important thing to keep in mind during the Upright Rows is that if you're rounding your back, you're not getting your core workout, which is especially intense when you do this pose correctly. So sit up straight! This is the kind of pose where sitting on a blanket can be helpful.

Boat with a Burn

This is a tough one, which is why it comes a little later in your Flat Belly Yoga! Workout, after you have developed some core strength. On its own, the Boat pose is challenging enough. But once you add in weights and start lowering down and coming back up again, there is nothing better for your core.

Warrior 1 and Warrior 2 with Weights

Not only are the Warrior poses good for feeling strong and tall, they are a good foundation on which to build additional exercises. When you're in a Warrior

mat motivation
My Most Difficult Pose

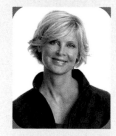 When I first got into yoga, I had been a long-distance runner for years and stretching my hips was always an issue for me. The Cobbler pose, which we will do in our Core+ Yoga workout, stretches your lower back, hips, and inner thighs. This pose in particular has always been challenging for me. Even today after years of practice, I still say that I love Cobbler pose and I hate it at the same time. It's tough, but it will develop your core strength, so you might have a love-hate relationship with it, too. There are poses that just click for me and are easy right away. (This may also be the case for you.) Most of the power poses that improve strength and flexibility, like Warrior 1 and Warrior 2, were always very easy for me. As you begin your workout, you'll begin to notice which poses are easy for you and which require more focus. So don't worry if everything doesn't immediately click for you—it didn't for me at first, either.

pose, your hands are free, so you have the ability to introduce variations that involve your upper body. Part of our goal with Yoga for Your Core and the Core+ Yoga workouts is to build lean muscle mass. Once you get to Warrior 1 or Warrior 2, everything you do from there builds muscle, especially with the addition of weights. It's an amazing workout.

Lat Rows

This stretch doesn't just work your basic core muscles, it also goes to town on your lats. (Those are the muscles across the top of your back.) The Flat Belly Yoga! Workout is designed to address all areas of your core, which—don't forget—is from your hips to your shoulders. Doing your lat rows will give you a beautiful back. (You may find that people will start asking if you're a swimmer!)

Cobbler with Chest Flies

Cobbler pose is a great hip opener. Sometimes you might have a hard time staying in the pose, but just like with Upright Rows, you have to sit up straight when you're doing it. By doing so, you will tap into your core strength.

Dead Bug with Chest Press

This is a pose that gets redefined by the addition of weights. In a traditional yoga practice, it's a relaxing stretch. But in a Core+ Yoga workout, this version requires work, and it definitely flattens your belly. It's a great pose to work your lower belly and to flatten out your abs.

The Core+ Yoga 30-Minute Workout

We will really bump it up with the Core+ Yoga 30-Minute Workout, which takes place in the last week of your 4-week program. It is the ultimate Core+ Yoga Workout, incorporating more challenging balancing poses like Warrior 3 to test how far you've come. By the time you get to this challenging workout, you and your core will be ready to take it to the next level.

Yoga and Style

Yoga has a lot of different styles, which I will share with you below, just in case you want to try a yoga class after finishing your Flat Belly Yoga! Workout. I hope this book does inspire you to continue doing yoga, whether it's continuing with your Core+ Yoga workouts, following along with a yoga DVD, or if you want to be more social, joining a class at a gym or a yoga studio. There are a lot of ways to include yoga as part of your fitness routine.

Flat Belly Yoga! comes out of my belief that yoga should be available to everyone. If you're not interested in or don't feel at home with chanting *om*, using long Sanskrit names to refer to poses, or the lifestyle that you may associate with yoga, that's okay. I'm offering you a practical guide to yoga. My goal is to make yoga more inclusive and accessible, so that's what *Flat Belly Yoga!* is about.

If someone tells you that there's only one way to practice yoga, they are wrong. There are at least a dozen different schools of yoga that are popular in the United States, all coming from the same tradition but with different practices.

If you're interested, here's a short guide to some of the different yoga styles and what you could expect if you were to take a class.

Hatha Yoga—*Hatha yoga* is a term that goes back to the 11th century. Today it is sometimes used as a catchall term for yoga that focuses on physical exercise. If a yoga studio doesn't say it teaches any particular kind of yoga, it probably teaches hatha yoga.

Iyengar Yoga—A form of hatha yoga created in the 1970s by B. K. S. Iyengar. Iyengar yoga is known for using props such as blocks, straps, and blankets. It's a great class for beginners or if you are dealing with an injury. This was the style of yoga I started with back in the '80s.

Sivananda Yoga—Follows the teachings of Swami Sivananda, as brought to the West by his disciple Swami Vishnudevananda. Vishnudevananda came to the United States in 1957, making this style of practice an important part of yoga's first wave of popularity outside India. There are now Sivananda yoga centers in every major city in the U.S.

Bikram Yoga—You might have heard of "hot yoga." Bikram yoga studios are heated to 105 degrees Fahrenheit. It was started in the 1970s by Bikram Choudhury. Bikram yoga is a set series of 26 poses. If you "like it hot," this is the class to go to. One of my first yoga conferences as a teacher was at a Bikram yoga expo held in downtown Los Angeles.

Ashtanga Yoga—Ashtanga Vinyasa yoga or Ashtanga yoga is a system of yoga popularized by K. Pattabhi Jois. The class is a series of poses that takes about an hour and a half to 2 hours to complete. Probably not the best place to start if you're a beginner since it's a pretty intense practice.

Kundalini Yoga—Kundalini yoga is entirely focused on the breath. If you take a Kundalini class, you'll spend much more time doing breathing exercises than moving through poses. But that might work for you.

Yoga has come a long way. What used to have the reputation of being just for the chosen few, those who could wrap themselves into pretzels or for the extreme yogi, has now become accessible to everyone and with a variety of styles to choose from. In fact, when I started YAS Fitness Centers, I created my own style of yoga called Yoga for Athletes® that caters to athletic types, also known as inflexible people. I designed *Flat Belly Yoga!* to be the gateway for you to get a taste of yoga. Just a little exposure, and if you find after the 32-day Flat Belly Yoga! program that you are thinking yoga is for you, you can explore all of the options available to you.

At this point, you've gotten a taste of the benefits of a yoga-based workout program and a sense of what's in store for you in the yoga part of your Flat Belly Yoga! Workout. But you're also going to be incorporating some cardio in the form of Heart Walks (see Chapter 3 on page 29) as well as strength training by adding weights to your yoga routine. So let's take a closer look at the importance of weight training in Chapter 2.

PLAY IT SAFE If you have any medical issues, always check with your doctor before you start a new exercise program.

A FLAT BELLY YOGA
SUCCESS STORY

Zoe Shepherd

Age: 42

Pounds lost:

7.5

in 32 days

All-over inches lost:

20.5

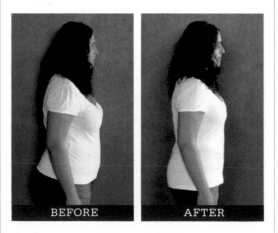

BEFORE · AFTER

"Yoga is absolutely a great way to lose weight. This is something I did not realize before starting the program," admits Zoe Shepherd. Before beginning the Flat Belly Yoga! Workout, Zoe had refused to even step foot into a yoga studio. Like a lot of people, Zoe was turned off by the idea of yoga, thinking it just wasn't right for her. "I had tried it previously and felt intimidated by the traditional yoga classes. Quite frankly, I felt it just wasn't my thing."

But when Zoe's current workout program stalled, she knew it was time to try something new. After hearing about the Flat Belly Yoga! Workout, she decided to give it a try. "With this program, the yoga feels targeted toward regular people who want to be healthy, get fit, and, if need be, lose weight," she says.

And now, after feeling more energized and seeing the physical benefits it brings, she's the first to say how much she enjoys practicing yoga. "I have become a total addict to yoga, which is a complete surprise to me."

In the beginning of the program, she was unable to hold a number of the yoga poses without feeling that she was going to collapse. But Zoe worked at it every day and eventually found herself holding the poses longer and longer. "I realized that the strength to hold the plank pose doesn't necessarily come from your arms and shoulders, like I thought, but from your core," she states. "I can absolutely feel a major difference in my core. I am physically feeling much stronger."

Yoga has also helped Zoe with her lower-back issues. The pain she was experiencing has disappeared since starting the program. "Yoga is the only change I made to my exercise routine," she says. "And since my lower-back pain has improved, this has led me to believe that it was because of yoga," says Zoe, noting that her sleep has improved as well.

Another perk? Zoe lost a total of 20.5 inches in 32 days. "I dropped at least one clothing size and I started to fit back into my old clothes!" And she wasn't the only one who noticed. By Week 3, everyone around her began telling her how great she looked.

Looking back, Zoe admits that over the years of trying many different exercise routines, the Flat Belly Yoga! Workout has been the one program she was able to continue. And her only regret is not having tried yoga sooner.

Even though she loved the feeling of completing the program, Zoe didn't stop her workouts after the 32 days were over. She maintained her workouts and has lost another 8 pounds. She is even on track to meet her goal of losing 25 pounds by the end of the year. "Now, I really look forward to doing yoga," she says. "It's physically challenging and I am really enjoying the feeling of getting stronger each time I do it. This exercise routine is totally addicting— I don't want to stop!

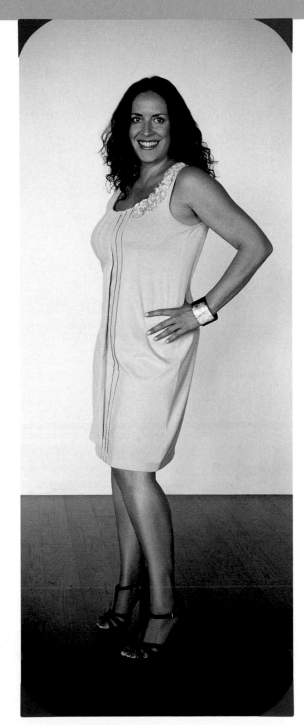

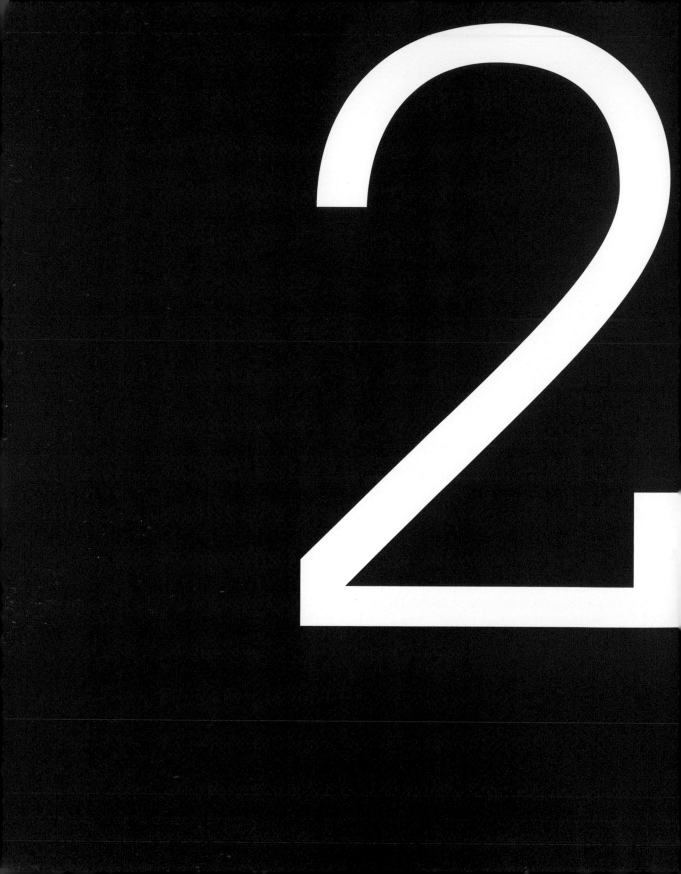

USING WEIGHTS

Weight training, also known as strength or resistance training, is an essential component of the Flat Belly Yoga! Core+ workouts. Studies have shown that by adding muscle mass, your body will burn more calories more efficiently, slimming you *and your belly* down in the process. Weight training, along with specific yoga poses designed to slim, tone, and flatten your belly, will kick your metabolism into high gear.

Using weights increases your muscle mass and strength, which also increases your fat-burning potential. It also raises your basal metabolic rate, or BMR, which is the number of calories you burn at rest per day.[1]

A yoga routine that incorporates weights is called a yoga-hybrid workout. You begin to see all the physical benefits of traditional yoga—such as strength, balance, and flexibility—a lot faster when you add weights. And each time you do the Core+ workouts, you will notice an increased sense of well-being along with a flatter and more toned belly.

Adding weights to straightforward yoga poses allows you to supercharge your workout and do it in less time. Resistance training combined with yoga also helps strengthen your core, which contributes to a flatter belly.

Getting Started

If you haven't used weights before, Core+ Yoga is a good place to start. Any form of strength training enhances your health, speeds up weight loss, and helps to flatten your belly. You may have tried yoga or weight training separately in the past, but combining them is a dynamic duo designed to target your belly. Yoga will tone and tighten your core, and holding the weights will build muscle mass and boost your metabolism.

Assuming you have little to no background in yoga or weight training, I will be breaking down the poses in basic terms so you can easily understand them. To begin, the 4-Day Jump Start, or Yoga for Your Core Workout, contains yoga moves without the use of weights. Instead, you will actually be using your own body weight as a strength-training tool. (It's important to learn the poses before adding weights in order to reduce your risk of injury.) So after you have practiced the yoga poses for 4 days, adding weights will be easier because doing yoga won't be a completely new concept.

I know getting started with strength training can be confusing. (How many sets and reps? How much weight? What types of weights should I buy?) I'm going to take away the confusion with a very straightforward and practical yoga-with-weights program.

The Terms: If you're picking up weights for the first time, here are some strength-training basics. The word *rep* is short for *repetition*. For example, each time you lift and lower a dumbbell, that's one rep. A specific number of reps is called a *set*.

Your Weights: Dumbbells. Don't be afraid of weights—you won't get big, bulky muscles. But you will get stronger and firmer faster than if you didn't incorporate them into your yoga routine. For the best results, the weight you choose should be heavy enough that by your last rep, you feel that you can't do any more while maintaining good form. I generally recommend one set of 3-pound weights (or 5-pound weights if you're a guy). They might feel light at the beginning. But don't worry—after a few reps you will definitely start to notice the difference. And lots of reps with lighter weights are just as effective at building up muscle as heavier ones. And some studies have shown that weight training at a lower intensity, but with more repetitions, may even be *more* effective for building muscle than lifting heavy weights.[2]

No Pain, No Gain—No Way!: If you're accustomed to workouts that leave you close to tears, you'll be happy to know that the Core+ workouts require no such sacrifice. We have a different rule of thumb: If it hurts, don't do it! The mantra *no pain, no gain* simply does not apply here.

Buying Weights: There are lots of brands out there, so don't get overwhelmed. The most important thing is to buy what you need to get started, which is a set of dumbbells. Take into consideration the durability and comfort of the weights (make sure the grips are comfortable). You can find weights at any sporting goods store. You can also purchase them online.

Why Muscle Up?

If you want to lose fat or change your body (i.e., flatten your belly), one of the most important things you can do is add weights to your workout. Aerobic exercise is also important, which is why we will be adding a walking program to the Flat Belly Yoga! Workout later in the book. But when it comes to changing how your body looks, using weights with yoga wins hands down.

If you've been "resistant" to trying resistance training, it may motivate you to know that lifting weights can help raise your metabolism. Muscle mass burns *seven times* more calories than fat—so the more muscle you have, the more calories you'll burn all day. It also strengthens bones, which is especially important for women (see the Weights and Osteoporosis section on page 22). Lifting weights obviously makes you stronger, which helps you avoid injuries by improving your coordination and balance. Plus, adding muscle increases your energy, which will make you more active throughout the day. And it'll make everyday tasks easier to do, too.

Here's another benefit of strength training: When you start to add muscle tone, it will increase your self-confidence. When you are toned, strong, and healthy, you feel better about yourself. What could be wrong with that?

Adding muscle mass is also extremely important as we get older. Starting around age 30, we start to lose about half a pound of muscle per year—a phenomenon known as *sarcopenia*. That's the primary reason we gain weight as we get older: With less muscle we burn fewer calories. And decreasing muscle mass also makes you weaker. Ordinary tasks, such as getting out of a chair or climbing the stairs, become more difficult. As a result, you start to move less—further contributing to muscle loss and fat gain.[3]

Strength training preserves and even rebuilds the muscle you have lost, which is the key to burning fat. So not only will you slim down your belly—you'll also take a major step in maintaining your overall health.

MUSCLE AND BELLY FAT

Abdominal (visceral) fat is of particular concern because it's a key player in a variety of health problems—much more so than subcutaneous fat (the kind you can grasp with your hand). Visceral fat lies out of reach, deep within the abdominal cavity where it pads the spaces between our abdominal organs.

Visceral fat has been linked to metabolic disturbances and increased risk for cardiovascular disease and type 2 diabetes. In women, it is also associated with breast cancer and the need for gallbladder surgery.

How Do We Build Muscle?

When you challenge a muscle, you create microscopic tears in your muscle tissue. (Don't worry, this is actually good for you.) Your body then comes to the rescue and fills those crevices with protein, creating new muscle tissue. Replacing the tissue creates stronger muscles, making our bodies look firmer, tighter, and more toned.

Scientists are also learning that visceral fat pumps out immune system chemicals called *cytokines*—like tumor necrosis factor and interleukin-6—that can increase the risk of cardiovascular disease. These and other biochemicals are thought to have deleterious effects on cells' sensitivity to insulin, blood pressure, and blood clotting.[4]

The best way to get rid of this dangerous fat is to combine aerobic workouts with yoga and strength training—exactly what you're getting with the Flat Belly Yoga! Workout. Adding muscle will not only help you look better in your jeans, but it will also keep you healthier longer so you can fully enjoy your flat belly.

WOMEN AND MUSCLE

Weight training is good for everyone, but it's especially important for women: If you don't do something to maintain your muscle mass, you can lose up to a pound of muscle each year once you hit menopause. And when you lose muscle, you gain weight. None of us can afford that!

Later, I'll talk about the importance of weighing youself regularly (see Chapter 6 on page 73), but you can't completely rely on your scale for a true measure of health because muscle is denser than fat by about 18 percent. That means even as you are losing belly fat and building muscle, you may not necessarily be losing pounds. So here's the bottom line: The more fat you replace by adding muscle with your Core+ workouts, the more calories you will burn. (And if you replace 10 pounds of fat with 10 pounds of lean muscle, you'll burn an additional 25 to 50 calories every day without even trying!)

Now, maybe you're afraid that by building muscle you'll start to look like an actual muscle builder. But unless you quit your day job and spend the next few years doing nothing but heavy lifting, you have nothing to worry about. Women simply do not, and cannot, naturally produce as much testosterone as males do, which is the main hormone responsible for increasing muscle size. Testosterone levels in women are typically only 5 percent to 10 percent of those in men.

The truth is that once you start to add muscle, you will begin to become lean. That's especially true if you are overweight, because the fat will turn into muscle. If you still don't believe me, picture a friend or co-worker with nice muscle tone and think of how attractive she looks. I guarantee that she got it through strength training. And I promise that if you add strength training to your yoga workout, you can achieve that same attractive muscle tone.

Weight training for women has never been more popular. That's why millions of women are doing it—and because they know it will help give them the flat belly they desire.

WEIGHTS AND OSTEOPOROSIS

Women begin losing bone mass in their mid-thirties—a loss that accelerates as they enter menopause, putting them at risk for osteoporosis.

What exactly is osteoporosis? It is the thinning of bone tissue and loss of bone density. One out of five women over the age of 50 develops osteoporosis, which can lead to accidental breaks and spontaneous fractures (when bones break for no apparent reason). Both of these types of fractures are harder to heal as women get older because there is less bone to knit the fracture back together. Bone loss also leads to spinal curvature, which—in addition to being uncomfortable—makes it impossible to stand straight and ultimately causes the belly to stick out.

Here's the good news: By adding weight training to your workout routine, you can significantly lessen your chance of developing bone disease. In fact, weight training is one of the primary recommendations for avoiding osteoporosis.

When a bone is stressed, either by muscular contractions or other methods of mechanical force, it begins a process of manufacturing protein molecules, which are deposited in the spaces between bone cells.[5] Strength training triggers this process by stretching and pulling muscles and tendons, thereby increasing bone density and reducing the risk of osteoporosis.

Among its many health benefits, weight-bearing and muscle-strengthening exercise can improve agility, strength, posture. and balance, which may reduce the risk of falls. The National Osteoporosis Foundation strongly endorses life-long physical activity at all ages, both for osteoporosis prevention and overall health, as benefits are lost when the person stops exercising. If you already have osteoporosis, strength training can lessen its impact. But be sure to check with your doctor before starting any exercise program.

OTHER BENEFITS OF STRENGTH TRAINING

Yes, we all want the flat belly that weight training can help us achieve. But adding muscle will change your life for the better in many ways:

You'll sleep better. People who do strength training regularly are less likely to struggle with insomnia. In a study conducted at Tufts University, 32 elderly men and women, described as slightly to moderately depressed, participated in either a 10-week strength-training program or a control group. The exercise group completed three strength-training sessions each week. At the end of the study, the strength-training group reported significant improvement over the control group in both quality of sleep and quality of life.[6]

You'll improve your balance. This may not be a concern now, but problems with balance can be a major health risk as we get older. As people age, poor balance and flexibility contribute to falls and broken bones. These fractures can result in significant disability and, in some cases, fatal complications. Strengthening exercises, when done properly and through the full range of motion, increase a person's flexibility and balance. This decreases the likelihood and severity of falls. In fact, a study in New Zealand showed that women 80 years of age and older had a 40-percent reduction in falls with simple strength and balance training.[7]

You'll strengthen your tendons and ligaments. Strong ligaments prevent joint laxity and too much mobility, which can cause weak joints and muscles. To prevent weak ligaments, try doing strength training daily to maintain ligament strength and normal range of motion.

You'll be less tired overall. Who doesn't want to have more energy? Well, weight training can help put a charge into your life. Approximately 25 percent of the US population experiences persistent fatigue symptoms. Impressively, 94 percent of the 70 randomized studies on exercise and fatigue show that exercise is more beneficial than drug or cognitive-behavioral interventions. In fact, a strength-training-only intervention results in the largest improvements in chronic fatigue.[8]

You'll improve your memory. I don't know about you, but a clearer mind and stronger memory are worth a lot to me—and weight training can help you attain both. Studies reveal that resistance training has been shown to improve several aspects of cognition in healthy older adults. One of the most profound effects of resistance training is the marked improvement in memory and memory-related tasks. Furthermore, resistance training can even improve your ability to solve problems, make decisions, and pay attention.[9]

You'll feel better about yourself. Sounds too good to be true—but it's not. Resistance training has been shown to improve self-esteem in healthy younger and older adults as well in cancer, cardiac rehabilitation, and depression patient populations.[9]

You'll reduce your risk of getting diabetes. Weight training lessens your chance of developing diabetes because lean muscle tissue helps your body metabolize blood sugar. Exercise helps reduce abnormal blood glucose by using it from the blood and muscle as fuel. It also makes the body more insulin sensitive and efficient at storing glucose in a form called *glycogen* in muscle and the liver.

Strength training has a particular role to play because when we lift or push weights, the main fuel used is that stored as muscle glucose. Building extra muscle also provides us with a larger storage area for glucose, so the combination of these two factors—increased muscle and regular emptying of these

mat motivation
How I Discovered Weights

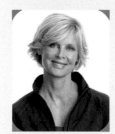

To be honest, I was never a "weights person." I was very sporty—I loved running, biking, swimming, and tennis, but I never incorporated weights into my workouts.

However, I have been doing yoga for a very long time. I started after I was hit by a car during a bicycle race. I used yoga as a recovery technique.

When I reached my fifties, students began asking me how to incorporate weight training into their workout regimen. So I came up with a program that incorporates weights with yoga. It was a fast way to build muscle tone—you can even see a difference after just a few workouts.

And I have to say that I love using weights with yoga to tone and flatten my belly (especially when I have a photo shoot coming up!). But you don't have to wait until a week before bathing-suit season to begin. Once you start combining yoga and weights, you'll always be ready for your close-up.

muscle stores—improves the body's glucose processing, a factor crucial in preventing and managing type 2 diabetes.[10]

You'll lower your cholesterol. We know that exercise can decrease cholesterol. But weight training, specifically, has been shown to be especially effective.

Research has consistently demonstrated that low concentrations of total cholesterol and low-density lipoprotein cholesterol (LDL-C), along with high levels of high-density lipoprotein cholesterol (HDL-C), are associated with a decrease in coronary heart disease. Also, several investigators have reported favorable changes in blood lipids and lipoproteins following a strength-training routine.

You'll look younger with your clothes off. Following a regular strength-training routine that creates more supportive muscle tone will help you firm sagging skin, giving your body a youthful appearance.[15]

You'll reverse the aging process at a cellular level. Weight training doesn't just help you look younger—it actually inhibits the aging process. Studies have shown that strength training twice a week on nonconsecutive days slows the aging process at the gene level. Furthermore, the gene expressions of the resistance-trained older participants demonstrated characteristics similar to those of the younger group.[11]

You'll minimize the appearance of cellulite. By building compact muscle, you will smooth out lumpy lower body fat.

Wayne L. Westcott, PhD, fitness researcher and author of *No More Cellulite*, designed a cellulite reduction program to test the effects of exercise on cellulite. This program was performed 3 days a week and included a 20-minute strength-training program along with 20 minutes of aerobic exercise. When compared with the control group, whose exercise was limited to only steady-state cardiovascular exercise, those who strength trained changed their body composition and reduced the appearance of cellulite. And those who performed only aerobic exercise lost weight but did not show a measurable difference in body composition or in the appearance of cellulite.[12]

PLAY IT SAFE If you get tired while using your weights, just put them down and do the Core+ Yoga Workout without them. Remember that you are in control of your workout and you need to listen to your body.

A FLAT BELLY YOGA
SUCCESS STORY

Robert Williams

Age: 45

Pounds lost:

21

in 32 days

All-over inches lost:

22

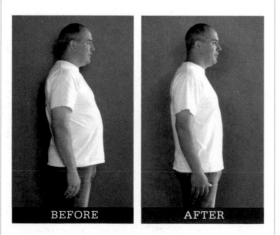

BEFORE | AFTER

66 I had not really worked out for 5 years when I began this program," admits Robert Williams, whose wife, Nicole, convinced him to try the Flat Belly Yoga! Workout. "My wife had been asked to be a participant, and she asked me if I wanted to do the program with her. We have three small children, including an 8-month-old, so she was excited to try to work off her baby weight." Seeing this as an opportunity to spend some quality time with his wife, Robert decided to give the program a chance.

When he first began the program, the 45-year-old father says he was out of shape. "During the first few days, I could barely sit up straight or do any of the poses," he says. "And as far as bending down and touching my toes . . . it was more like touching my knees!" But by the end of the first week, he began to notice that his flexibility had improved and he was able to put more effort into his workouts.

He also said goodbye to his daily aches and pains. "Since I began the program, I have not had a single headache. My back has been a problem for a few years, and now it feels great. All of the little aches and pains of aging have gone away because of the workouts and the weight loss."

In fact, when Robert weighed himself after the first week on the Flat Belly Yoga! Workout, he found that he had lost an astonishing 10 pounds! The following week, he discovered he'd lost another 5 pounds. "At the end of the third week, I did not even weigh myself," he says. "I didn't care anymore about how much weight I lost because I felt so good! That was when I really realized this plan was working for me."

Having tried numerous workout routines in the past, Robert states that this is the only program he's been able to maintain because he now looks forward to working out. "It's funny because I originally decided to do the program because I thought it would be fun to do something like this with my wife," he says. "But we lead a very busy life and ended up only doing one workout together on a Sunday morning. The rest of the time, I would do the yoga-with-weights workout at home alone after my family went to bed. And I love that time now—I get 1 free hour a day all to myself!"

Robert hasn't yet reached his goal weight, but he's optimistic about his future health, saying he plans to continue his Flat Belly Yoga! Workouts. When asked how he feels about his belly now, he smiles and says, "I like it, but ask me again in 32 days. I cannot believe what can happen in 32 days. **"**

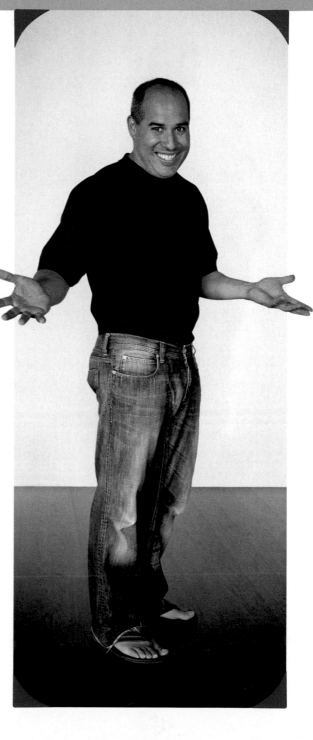

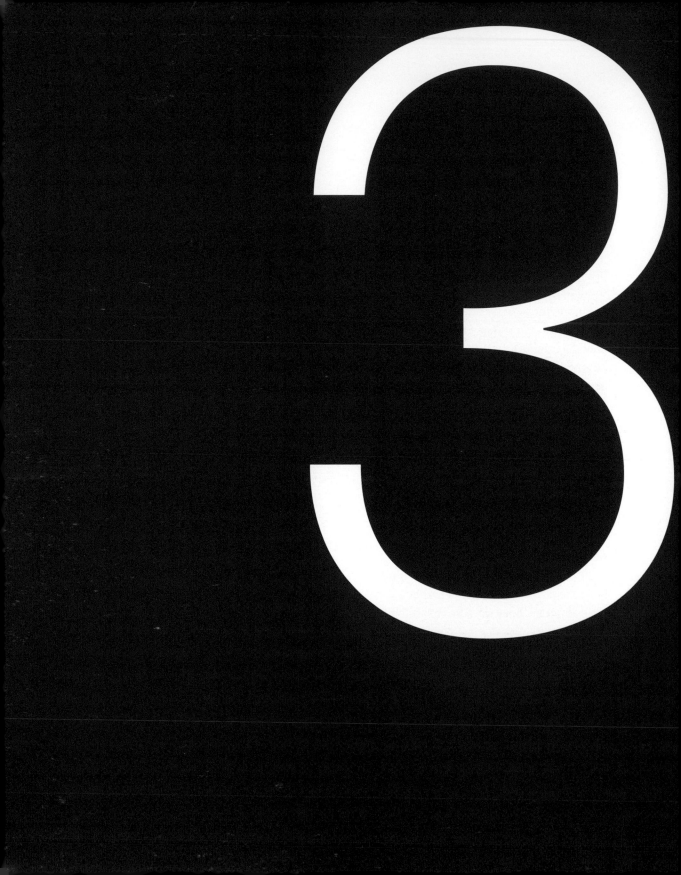

THE BENEFITS OF WALKING

Why walking? Well, simply put, walking powers weight loss by getting your heart pumping. According to a recent study, aerobic exercise is your best bet when it comes to losing that dreaded belly fat.[1] And in another study, researchers from the Washington University School of Medicine in St. Louis reported that walking just 45 minutes just a few times resulted in weight loss—primarily from the belly area.[2]

If that's not enough to convince you that walking should be your go-to cardio, let's take a look at some other health benefits.

Health Benefits of Walking

With each step you take, you'll be moving toward a flat belly. And you'll also be picking up a ton of other important health benefits along the way. Walking—that thing most of us learned to do around the age of 1—can improve the health of your heart, blood, bones, lungs, and even your mind. Does that sound a little too good to be true? Let's take a look at the science behind walking.

Walking is good for your overall health. It helps you stay strong and fit, manage your weight, and reduce the chance of developing type 2 diabetes, according to the Mayo Clinic.[3]

Walking can lead to healthier blood. The Mayo Clinic also notes that walking helps lower your low-density lipoprotein (LDL) cholesterol (also known as the "bad" cholesterol) while raising high-density lipoprotein (HDL) cholesterol (the "good" cholesterol). And it lowers your blood pressure, lessening the risk of heart disease and stroke.

Walking is good for your heart. Guess what this means? You can forget the phrase *no pain, no gain.* Research shows that regular, brisk walking is just as effective at reducing the risk of heart attacks as more vigorous exercise, such as jogging. So stroll with the confidence that you're getting the same health benefits as that runner down the street.

Walking strengthens your bones. Another benefit of walking is that it helps build bone density, even in postmenopausal women, who are at risk for bone density loss.[4] Walking can reduce your risk of injuries, such as a hip fracture, by as much as 50 percent. And adding yoga also improves stamina and balance, which will help you avoid falls.

Walking can improve your mental health. That's right—walking can actually keep your brain and mind healthier. If you need a natural stress reliever, put on those walking shoes. Walking can make you feel better by relieving stress and boosting your mood. Researchers at St. Louis University found that cardio exercise like walking improves mood and energy and can help prevent some anxiety and depression.[5] And according to a study in the

British Journal of Sports Medicine, a walking program provided faster relief than antidepressants in those suffering from depression.[6]

It can also help protect your brain from the impacts of aging, such as memory loss. A study at the University of California, San Francisco found that women over 65 who walked more experienced a lower age-related decline in memory on average. The researchers also found that a walking program actually helped slow or halt the progression of Alzheimer's disease.[7]

Walking helps you sleep better. Like other forms of exercise, a regular walking routine will improve the quality of your sleep, which helps fend off stress, minor depression, and other mental challenges. A study by the Fred Hutchinson Cancer Research Center in Seattle found that women who walked for an hour a day experienced relief from insomnia.[8]

All you have to do to gain all of the benefits listed above is follow the Flat Belly Yoga! Heart Walk routines, named for their ability to get your heart pumping. Sounds pretty simple, right? (Don't worry, I'll show you how to do these walks in Chapter 6, starting on page 80.)

The Heart Walks are an important part of the Flat Belly Yoga! Workout. And you will be working your way up to walking 6 days a week by the end of the program. And here's the best part about walking: It's effective *and* it's easy. It's not something we have to learn to do in order to get a great fat-burning workout. It's just one foot in front of the other. Yes, there are a few tips and techniques that I'll cover in Chapter 6 to help you get on your way, but you already have the foundation. It is also easy to fit walking into a workout and stay with it. Most of us can do it anytime and pretty much anywhere.

Your Heart Walks are divided into two categories: Fat Blast walks and Calorie Torch walks. Fat Blast walking consists of steady-paced walking, which is guaranteed to burn off belly fat. Calorie Torch walking involves intervals of fast-paced walking and moderate-paced walking. We call it the Calorie Torch because this type of interval exercise has been shown to keep metabolism high well after you've come back from that walk—meaning you will continue burning belly fat all day long.

Importance of Speed and Intensity

Nothing good comes without effort. If you're going to lose your belly fat, and if you want to experience all the benefits of walking we just discussed, we need to get your walk to the point where you're breathing heavy and your heart is really pumping. A Heart Walk is not a leisurely stroll in the park. It's an aerobic exercise designed to burn calories and attack your belly fat.

Luckily, there is no mystery to exercising effectively. As long as you are following your program, the more effort you put in, the more calories you will burn and the more benefits you will see. There's a reason we call it a *work*out!

Some people use walking as a form of meditation. But for the Flat Belly Yoga! Workout, we need to get your heart rate up to burn fat. So taking gentle, peaceful walks isn't the purpose of your Heart Walks. You can still do some meditative practices while walking—just make sure you don't relax into a slower pace. While keeping up the pace needed for your workout, choose to focus on your breath, footsteps, or even the sound of the wind. Let any busy thoughts float away until after you've finished your workout.

You also might want to try and visualize your flat belly. Or sometimes it's good to let off a little steam as you walk. Think about whatever it is that's upsetting you and walk even faster. This will allow you to get it out of your head. And by the end of your walk, you'll feel relieved and rejuvenated. I like to do this—running a business can be stressful. I like the fact that I can go for a walk and leave the stress behind for a few minutes while I blow off steam and blow off calories at the same time.

Mixing It Up

Throughout this exercise program, you will be alternating your walks. From one day to the next, you will be moving back and forth between Fast Blast walks and Calorie Torch walks. And within the Calorie Torch walks, you will be alternating intervals of fast and medium-brisk paces.

This does a few things for you. First, alternating the type of walks allows you to receive the benefits of multiple types of workouts. Second, training in intervals maximizes the impacts—and the benefits—of your workout program.

You can also mix up the routes you take to keep yourself interested and engaged. I'm a creature of habit, so I like to use the same route every day. I don't have to think about where I'm going—I just go! But if you feel yourself becoming bored with your walking routine, just look for a change of scenery.

Comfort is a factor, too. You might choose a route with shade on particularly sunny days, and save the path with no cover for a cloudy or overcast day. (But remember to always use sunscreen.)

Mixing in routes with different terrains and challenges can push your body and increase the impact of your workouts, especially if you are introducing some slope into your journey. Going up and down is a quick and easy way to get a challenging cardio workout—and a great leg workout, too. There are different types of such walks, from climbing steps to walking up your favorite hill or ski slope, depending where you live. In fact, stadium steps have become popular places to get a great workout while enjoying the social aspects of exercise.

WHAT IS INTERVAL TRAINING?

Interval training is built upon alternating short, high-intensity bursts of speed with slower, recovery phases within a single workout. Interval workouts are often used to train professional athletes, and these workouts can be highly structured and complex. But I've included an easy-to-follow interval workout for your Heart Walks because it's the most effective—not only for your heart, but also for losing weight.

Interval training is an essential component of your Heart Walks because it burns more calories than a steady-paced walk. According to the American College of Sports Medicine, more calories are burned in short, high-intensity exercise.[9] If you are counting the calories you've burned, high-intensity exercises like fast-paced walking intervals are better than long, slow-endurance exercise. However, there are risks inherent in high-intensity training, so it's important to know both the benefits and dangers.

- Warm up before starting your interval walking program.
- Assess your current conditioning and set training goals that are within your ability.
- Start slowly. In general, longer intervals provide better results.
- Keep a steady but challenging pace throughout the interval.
- Build the number of repetitions over time.
- Bring your heart rate down during the rest interval.
- To improve, increase intensity or duration but not both at the same time.
- Initially train on a smooth, flat surface to ensure even effort.

Moving Forward

The benefits of the Flat Belly Yoga! Workout increase with time, and this is especially true of your walking workouts. There will be 6 Heart Walks every week—and it's important to push yourself to complete them every day. When you are balancing work, family, and other obligations, obstacles will come up. Sometimes it won't be possible to complete a day's walk. It happens. Just make sure you dedicate yourself to getting back on your feet and out on your next walk as soon as possible. If you miss 2 days of walks, don't let the discouragement lead you to miss a third. Instead, look at that third day as your next opportunity to get back on track to a flat belly!

Remember, something is better than nothing. If you can absolutely only spare 20 minutes when you had planned a 45-minute workout, really push yourself to get a good 20-minute walk in. Don't settle for zero because you couldn't complete the total scheduled time.

You should also have backup plans for your walks in case you encounter other disruptions. Is it too cold and rainy for a healthy walk? You can go to a mall. Not only are they temperature controlled, they're also full of distractions (think window-shopping and people-watching) to make your walking time go by more quickly. Did a business trip land you in an unfamiliar city where you don't feel safe? See if there's a treadmill in your hotel or walk up and down the stairway in your building.

Walking Buddies

When it comes to walking, finding a buddy—whether it be a person or "man's best friend"—can enhance your performance and actually make you healthier. And a recent study published in the *Journal of Personality and Social Psychology* found that walking with your dog can actually be better for you than walking with your human friend because dogs are better at helping us deal with stress.[10] And that may be part of the reason that exercising with them can improve your health more effectively than exercising alone or with another person. (Just make sure to save your intervals for days when Fido can't join you—it could be too much for him if he's not used to them.)

 If you are walking at night, you might want to bring a dog or a "walk buddy." See "Rules for Walking" on page 66 for more safety tips.

A FLAT BELLY YOGA
SUCCESS STORY

Nicole Williams

Age: 40

Pounds lost:

2

in 32 days

All-over inches lost:

8.5

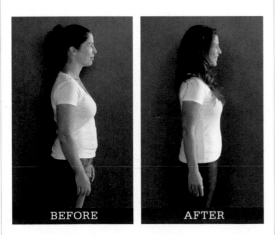

BEFORE   AFTER

"I have three daughters under 5 years old, so I haven't had my body to myself for nearly 6 years," states Nicole Williams. "After back-to-back pregnancies and nursing, my body felt flabby and weak. I hadn't exercised regularly for years, so I was a bit terrified of jumping back in at full speed, but I knew I needed to do something."

Since she was still breastfeeding at the time, Nicole didn't try the Flat Belly Yoga! Workout with the goal of restricting calories or losing weight. Instead, it was about finally making some time for herself to workout again and tone her belly. "I work 40 to 50 hours a week and also care for three young children, so finding the time was equally as terrifying as finding the stamina."

So between not exercising for years and having an extremely limited schedule, Nicole was concerned about how she was going to incorporate the workout into her lifestyle. Realizing that her only option was to schedule early morning workouts, Nicole woke up at 5:00 a.m. every morning to exercise. Her husband, Robert (featured in Chapter 2), looked after their children so that Nicole could focus on herself. She would then return the favor. "Once I would get home from work in the evenings, I wanted to give my daughters my full attention, so that's when my husband would do his workout."

Soon after beginning the routine, the 40-year-old began to notice some positive changes taking place. Not only did she gain more energy after each workout, but she also noticed that she was feeling stronger immediately after beginning the program. "I was reinvigorated," she says. "And since I am always giving to my children, my work, my husband, and the community, I looked forward to that one hour in the morning when I was dedicated to my physical health."

Nicole's favorite part of the program was having some quiet time in the morning when she could go on walks by herself. "The Heart Walks were tough in the beginning, but I ended up loving it because of the results I was seeing."

Even though she wasn't trying to lose weight, Nicole says she did notice a difference in her body. By the last week of the program, most of her maternity and post-maternity clothes were too large for her smaller frame. And there was an added bonus when she tried on her pre-pregnancy clothes: the pants that she wore before her pregnancies finally fit again. "My belly now feels tighter, slimmer, and healthier. After 6 years of taking care of my babies and not my body, this was exactly the challenge I needed to get back the focus on my health."

And now that she's focused on her well-being, Nicole isn't looking back. "I do have a ways more to go—one month can't reverse back-to-back-to-back belly-stretching," she says. "After the 32 days, I saw a glimpse of the figure I had pre-mommyhood. I became much happier and much more confident than I used to be. I feel like the program was my running start to continue to get my body back. It's empowering because I learned that I can get my strength and my body back."

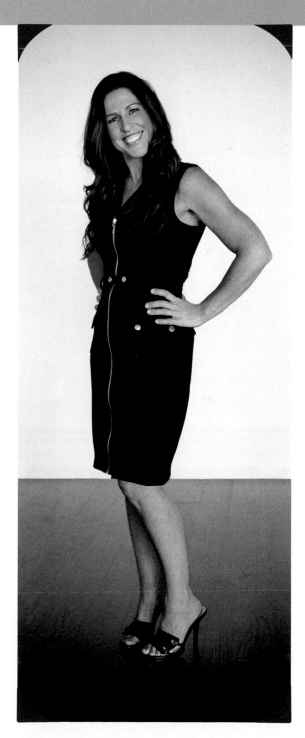

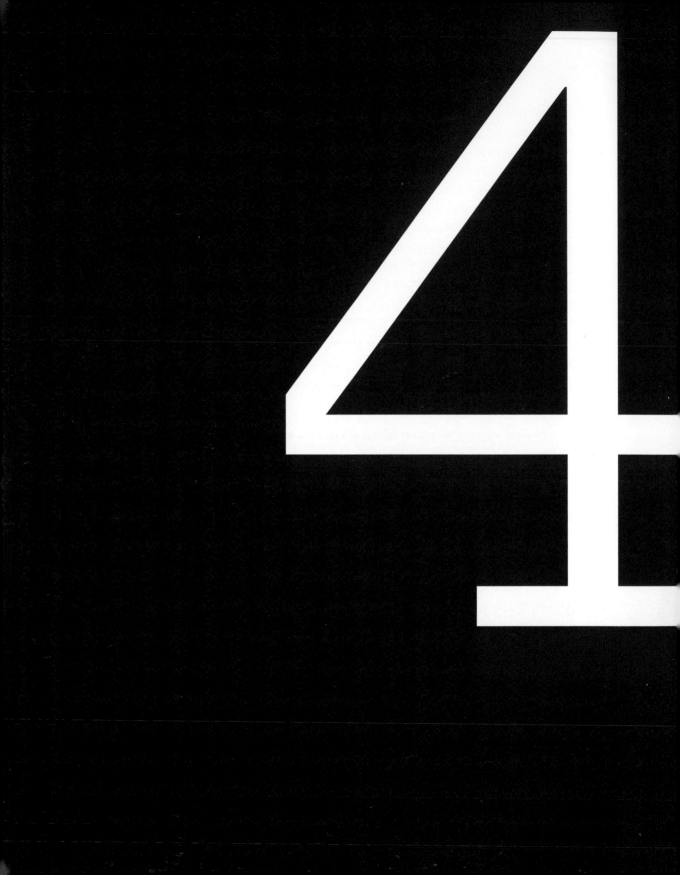

THE MIND-BELLY CONNECTION

When you look good, you feel better about yourself. And the Flat Belly Yoga! Workout makes you look good and feel good, which is why it won't be hard to stay with it once you begin the program. It's designed to deliver results you can see quickly—helping you to stay motivated and keep moving forward with your workouts.

A critical component to sticking with any exercise plan is learning to overcome stress, which may start in your mind but eventually works its way to your belly. So turn the page to read my suggestions for staying stress-free and on target with your goal.

Battling Stress and Anxiety

How's this for motivation? Working out delivers more than a flat belly—it helps to lower stress and anxiety, which in turn help us keep the belly fat off.

Research has shown that both stress and anxiety can interfere with efficient fat burning and lead to self-defeating behaviors. Many people deal with stress and anxiety by seeking comfort in food, often overeating and choosing unhealthy snacks as well as avoiding activity and skipping exercise.

Now, as you know, I'm a health and fitness expert. But sometimes even I turn to my comfort foods when I become stressed. (Chocolate cookies are my weakness. It's funny, because my students know that I love them, so they make them for me all the time. I have a student who is a flight attendant from Sweden, and she always brings me cookies when she returns from a trip. Yikes!) So I know it's hard to resist the temptation.

But that's the worst choice you can make—the right kind of exercise is actually the best medicine for stress. The Yoga for Your Core and Core+ workouts, with their basis in yoga poses and exercises, are as good at delivering stress relief as they are at strengthening your core. Both go a long way in helping you maintain a positive outlook that will improve your attitude, your ability to work out, and your ability to burn fat.

So all you need to get started is the right plan and the right attitude. Here's the good news: The right plan is in your hands right now. But the right attitude is up to you. Start working on it now, even as you read. Talk positively to yourself; learn how to be kinder to yourself. I know this is hard—I have issues with this, too. But it's time to change "I can't do this" into "I *can* do this!" After all, you've already chosen to do something about your belly fat and develop a healthier, happier you!

Think Positive Thoughts

When it comes to self-criticism, women are really tough on themselves. That's not to say that men are immune from this problem. But we women seem to have a critical self-talk loop going on in our brains. And most of us are worrywarts. The Flat Belly Yoga! program will help break your habit of self-criticism because anytime you have a negative thought during your workout, you'll be writing it down in your Flat Belly Yoga! Journal in Chapter 9 (see page 177). And after you write it down, I want you to change it into a positive one.

This doesn't mean negative thoughts will disappear completely, but it does mean you're taking control. When you focus on positive, factual information instead of negative, often overexaggerated, thoughts, you have more options and directions to go in. The most important fact to focus on as you adopt the Flat Belly Yoga! Workout into your daily regimen is that you are taking control of your situation. You have a plan that's effective and easy to follow—and with every step you're getting closer to your goals. So think positively! You've got a reason to be optimistic. And the great thing about optimism is that it's contagious—so you'll start to be more positive about other things, too.

Optimists also tend to experience less stress than pessimists or realists. Because they believe in themselves and their abilities, they expect good things to happen. They see negative events as minor setbacks to be easily overcome, and view positive events as evidence of further good things to come. So if you begin to believe in yourself, you'll start taking more risks and ultimately create more positive events in your life.[1]

A positive attitude can also get you over a hump if you've hit a plateau with your fitness and help take you to the next level. And it can help keep you motivated to maintain a regular exercise program, which has been proven to reduce stress and anxiety. It will also help you to get some rest. Getting a good night's sleep has been shown not only to help you burn fat more efficiently, but also to improve your state of mind, which will only make you want to work out more!

Get Your Groove On

Studies have shown that music may be the single best motivator for your workout. So make sure you find music that's right for you and the various steps and stages of your workouts.

(continued on page 44)

MOVE TO THE MUSIC

Looking for suggestions for music at the right beats per minute (BPM) for your Heart Walks? Here are some playlists that will get you moving (all approximately 20 minutes long):

Flat Belly Funk

Song: "Twenty-Five Miles"
Artist: Edwin Starr
Album: *25 Miles*
Time: 3:21

Song: "Word Up!"
Artist: Cameo
Album: *The Best of Cameo*
Time: 4:22

Song: "Early in the Morning"
Artist: The Gap Band
Album: *Gap Band IV*
Time: 3:57

Song: "I Feel for You"
Artist: Chaka Khan
Album: *I Feel for You*
Time: 5:46

Song: "Higher Ground"
Artist: Stevie Wonder
Album: *Innervisions*
Time: 3:42

Flat Belly Rock

Song: "Walk This Way"
Artist: Aerosmith
Album: *Toys in the Attic*
Time: 3:32

Song: "Feels Like the First Time"
Artist: Foreigner
Album: *Foreigner*
Time: 3:54

Song: "Hot Legs"
Artist: Rod Stewart
Album: *Foot Loose & Fancy Free*
Time: 5:15

Song: "Takin' Care of Business"
Artist: Bachman-Turner Overdrive
Album: *Bachman-Turner Overdrive II*
Time: 4:52

Song: "Dancing in the Street"
Artist: David Bowie and Mick Jagger
Album: *Best of Bowie*
Time: 3:22

Flat Belly Dance

Song: "Cream"
Artist: Prince
Album: *Diamonds and Pearls*
Time: 4:13

Song: "Don't Stop 'Til You Get Enough"
Artist: Michael Jackson
Album: *Off the Wall*
Time: 3:56

Song: "Move This"
Artist: Technotronic
Album: *Pump Up the Jam*
Time: 5:23

Song: "I Like the Way" (Radio Edit)
Artist: Bodyrockers
Album: *Bodyrockers*
Time: 3:20

Song: "Queen of the Night" (C.J's Single Edit)
Artist: Antonio "L.A." Reid, Babyface, Daryl Simmons, and Whitney Houston
Album: *Whitney—The Greatest Hits*
Time: 3:46

Flat Belly Old-School Hip-Hop

Song: "It's All Good"
Artist: MC Hammer
Album: *The Funky Headhunter*
Time: 4:14

Song: "Ice Ice Baby"
Artist: Vanilla Ice
Album: *To the Extreme*
Time: 4:31

Song: "Gettin' Jiggy Wit It"
Artist: Will Smith
Album: *Big Willie Style*
Time: 3:49

Song: "I Like to Move It"
Artist: Reel 2 Real
Album: *Monster Booty*
Time: 3:52

Song: "Push It"
Artist: Salt-N-Pepa
Album: *Hot, Cool & Vicious*
Time: 4:32

Choosing the right music is mostly about understanding a song's tempo or beats per minute (BPM). It's the easiest way to know if a song is a good match for your workout.

And in order to make your Heart Walk a true cardio workout, you have to move. You don't have to jog or race walk, but you do need to get your heart pumping.

The right music can help you set and keep a good pace. According to Costas Karageorghis, PhD, an associate professor of sports psychology at Brunel

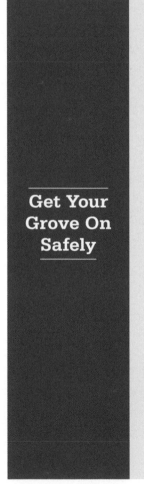

Get Your Grove On Safely

Don't pump it up all the way! You want the volume to be high enough for the energy to move you, but no higher. Headphones are so close to your ears that they can damage hearing much more quickly than speakers or live noise. You also want to be able to hear loud noises—like a honking car or a shouting biker—over your music. For these reasons, noise-blocking headphones are a bad idea out on the sidewalk.

Maintain your awareness. With your hearing partially blocked, you need to compensate by raising your awareness of what's happening around you. It helps to walk in a neighborhood that's familiar to you.

Look both ways. Headphones make it harder to hear cars and other vehicles approaching. Double-check traffic in both lanes before crossing the street. Take off your headphones before crossing busy or dangerous intersections. And don't jaywalk—it's dangerous and not worth the fine you could get if a cop catches you.

Stick to safe routes in view of others. Don't walk alone in unsafe or abandoned areas, especially at night. This is important common sense when planning any walks. But remember that earphones make it harder to hear approaching footsteps or cars and keep track of who's around you.

University in England, there is a science to choosing an effective exercise soundtrack.[2] By choosing a song with a BPM of 120 to 140, you'll set a pace that coincides with the range of most commercial dance music and many rock songs. It also roughly corresponds to the average person's heart rate during a routine workout. Just remember to pick music that makes you feel good and full of energy—you'll be surprised at how quickly the miles seem to fly by.

The Mind-Belly Connection

In the Flat Belly Diet!, the Mind-Belly Connection referred to your mind's connection, or lack thereof, with food. There are more emotional issues with eating than there are with exercise, which is good news for us! But there is still a Mind-Belly Connection when it comes to your mood or willingness to work out. For example, you might find yourself saying, "I don't have the energy to work out," or "I'm just too tired." Is that actually true? Or are you just not feeling very motivated?

Usually, when you don't have time or you feel tired and unmotivated to exercise, it's because of stress. Life can be stressful, I know. Work, kids, and even little things like deciding when to go shopping or pick up your dry cleaning can stress us out.

The great thing about yoga, and working out in general, is that it makes you happy by de-stressing your mind. I often hear comments from students that they're feeling frazzled. I get it: I run a fairly large company, and even though it's in the fitness industry, it's still work. And, like you, I have experienced times when I want to pull my hair out.

When it comes to stress, we have actual stress hormones, which are called *cortisol* and *adrenaline*. And if you don't keep these hormones in check, they can impair your memory and also raise your risk of depression and anxiety.

Luckily, when you work out, your serotonin levels rise in your brain, which makes you feel good and ultimately lowers stress. (I'm sure you have heard of a runner's high.) With a 20-minute workout you can boost your mood for as long as 12 hours.

GETTING STRESSED OUT

"I'm stressed out." I hear this all the time as one of the reasons people do not work out. People often not only miss workouts when they're stressed—they also eat more for comfort. It's a vicious cycle that we have to get out of. The sad thing about this is that working out really fights stress! Sometimes you just need to get out of the house, and going for a walk can actually make you feel better.

Aerobic exercise, like your Heart Walks, eases stress, while yoga emphasizes your breathing, which helps you relax. People who exercise—and I'm hoping that's you now—respond better to stress than those who don't exercise. Your blood pressure doesn't become as elevated when you experience stress, and your mood tends to stay more positive. Also, the more you exercise, and especially practice your yoga poses, the more in tune you will become with your body.

It's a good idea to keep track of your stressors—the things in your life that cause you stress. Recording these in your Flat Belly Yoga! Journal will help you become aware of what actually causes stress in your life. Once you have identified your stressors, you might be surprised to realize that it may just take minor adjustments to relieve a lot of the stress from your life.

THE SCIENCE OF STRESS

Stress is a term that is commonly used today but has become increasingly difficult to define. It shares, to some extent, common meanings in both the biological and psychological sciences. Stress typically describes a negative concept that can have an impact on our mental and physical well-being. But it's unclear what exactly defines stress and whether or not stress is a cause, an effect, or actually the process connecting the two. So while the science behind stress can be complicated, it's still good to know how it affects your body.

There are two types of stress: acute, which is short-term stress, and chronic, which is long-term. Can you already think of the things causing stress in your life? Long-term stress could come from a job, or a marriage, which you feel you can't leave. Acute stress results from things that just happened: Someone almost hit you in a car, or there was an emergency with a family member. In this case, your heart is racing. We often hear of this as a fight-or-flight response. It's your body's ancient way of preparing itself to deal with danger.

Stress starts with your central nervous system, which is responding to your thoughts. We also have the autonomic nervous system, which just functions on its own, meaning it works without you thinking about it. An example of this would be breathing. The autonomic nervous system has two parts: the sympathetic nervous system and the parasympathetic nervous system. The sympathetic nervous system activates what we described as the fight-or-flight response. The parasympathetic nervous system brings your body back to normal after experiencing stress. So here's what happens when your brain perceives a stressful situation:

The hypothalamus in your brain will send a message to your adrenal glands. Your adrenal glands release the hormones adrenaline and cortisol. I'm sure you have heard of adrenaline. It increases your heart rate, which will send extra blood to your brain. Your memory gets sharper and your body, especially your immune system, goes on high alert. Then your pupils will dilate, which causes your vision to become clearer.

Cortisol works on a different timetable. Its job is to help us replenish our body after the stress has passed, and it hangs around a lot longer. And it can remain elevated, which increases your appetite and ultimately drives you to eat more, according to Elissa S. Epel, PhD, a psychiatry professor at the University of California, San Francisco.

While this system works fine when our stress comes in the form of physical danger—when we really need to fight or flee, and then replenish—it doesn't serve the same purpose for today's garden-variety stressors.

According to Shawn M. Talbott, PhD, former director of the University of Utah Nutrition Clinic and author of *The Cortisol Connection*, we have a tendency to respond to stress by dwelling on our frustration and anger without expending the calories we would otherwise be if we were physically fighting our way out of danger. Furthermore, we have turned to eating as a way of coping and relieving stress.

In other words, since your neuroendocrine system doesn't know that you didn't fight or flee, it still responds to stress with the hormonal signal to replenish nutritional stores—which may make you feel hungry.[3]

When the immediate threat goes away, our parasympathetic nervous system kicks in, bringing our body back to normal—or at least it's supposed to. When we're under chronic stress—or when we feel stress all the time—what scientists call the normal "relaxation response" never begins and that hunger sensation doesn't subside.

CHRONIC STRESS

Chronic stress, as the term implies, is ongoing and doesn't stop. This is the stress we feel in a bad marriage, from work-related issues, or from dealing with aging parents. A number of my students are dealing with aging parents at the moment. As for me, I have a growing company with more than 100 employees, so I've been under chronic stress for about 11 years. Owning and running a business, even though it's based around the relaxing art of yoga, is still very stressful. I'm lucky that I am able to exercise for a living, which fights off those extra calories I may consume when I'm stressed out. Unfortunately, the longer your body is in "stress mode," the harder it is to turn it off.

Here are some physical signs of chronic stress:

- Headaches
- Diarrhea or constipation, frequent upset stomach
- Nausea, dizziness
- Chest pain, rapid heartbeat, or feeling like you can't catch your breath
- Feeling nervous or sad
- Feeling irritable and angry
- Having problems sleeping, insomnia or sleeping too much
- Lack of energy
- Fatigue, mental and/or physical
- Grinding your teeth
- Loss of sex drive
- Frequent colds, illness

REMEMBER CORTISOL?

Many of the symptoms above are caused by all the cortisol hanging around in our bodies. This is a powerful hormone. Prolonged high levels of cortisol in the bloodstream, which are associated with chronic stress, have been shown to have negative effects, such as:

- Impaired cognitive performance
- Suppressed thyroid function
- Blood sugar imbalances such as hyperglycemia
- Decreased bone density
- Decrease in muscle tissue
- Higher blood pressure
- Lowered immunity and inflammatory responses in the body, which cause slowed wound healing and other health consequences
- Increased abdominal fat, which is associated with a greater amount of health problems than fat deposited in other areas of the body.[4]

STRESS AND BELLY FAT

Being stressed all the time is no joke. It even leads to more belly fat. That's right: more belly fat. How? Chronic stress leads to more cortisol. And more cortisol leads to more fat—specifically belly fat.

Studies at Wake Forest University revealed that female monkeys suffering from higher stress had higher levels of visceral fat in their bodies. This suggests a possible cause-and-effect link between the two, wherein stress promotes the accumulation of visceral fat, which in turn causes hormonal and metabolic changes that contribute to heart disease and other health problems.

Why does that happen? It isn't just because cortisol makes you hungry, though that is part of it. It's also because that burst of adrenaline you get when you're exposed to stress tells your body to release insulin, the hormone your muscles need to draw energy from your bloodstream. Then, because your body expects to have used up all its energy, the cortisol that kicks in makes you crave fast-energy foods like sugars and carbs. That's why stress makes you crave food like ice cream or potato chips.

So now you have all this insulin and sugar floating around in your blood all the time. Your body responds to that by storing all that extra sugar as belly fat.

Non-overweight women who are vulnerable to the effects of stress are more likely to have excess abdominal fat and higher levels of the stress hormone cortisol, a study conducted at Yale University suggests. Cortisol affects fat distribution by causing fat to be stored centrally—around the organs.[4] And remember how in the Introduction we talked about how belly fat increases your risk of serious problems like Alzheimer's disease, stroke, diabetes, cancer, and heart disease? That's why we keep talking about the Mind-Belly Connection. Stress affects your mind, which goes right to your belly, and that hurts your whole body.

STRESS RELIEF AND WEIGHT LOSS

Lucky for us, this works both ways. If stress is a big part of what's giving us belly fat, then de-stressing can also be a big part of getting to a flat belly.

In a study by UCSF researchers published online in the *Journal of Obesity*, mastering simple mindful eating and stress-reduction techniques helped prevent weight gain even without dieting. And subjects who experienced the greatest reduction in stress lost the most belly fat.[5] So instead of stressing about your belly, get rid of your stress *to get rid of your belly.*

EXERCISE: STRESS RELIEVER

Exercise increases your overall health and your sense of well-being, which puts more pep in your step. And the Flat Belly Yoga! Workout has some direct stress-busting benefits.

The Heart Walks pump up your brain's feel-good endorphins. Although this is often called a runner's high, a fast-paced walk can also provide this same feeling.

In a way, your Heart Walks can also be moving meditations. After a walk or a Core+ Yoga workout, you'll often find that you've forgotten the irritations—or stresses—of the day, because you are only concentrating on your body's movements. As you begin to regularly shed your daily tensions through movement and physical activity, you may find that focusing on a single task—and the resulting energy and optimism—can help you remain calm and clear in any situation.

Biologically, exercise seems to give the body a chance to practice dealing with stress. It forces the body's physiological systems—all of which are involved in the stress response—to communicate much more closely than usual: The cardiovascular system communicates with the renal system, which communicates with the muscular system. And all of these are controlled by the central and sympathetic nervous systems, which also must communicate with each other. This workout of the body's communication system may be the true value of exercise; the more sedentary we get, the less efficient our bodies become in responding to stress.[6]

Exercise helps relieve stress in other ways, too. It can increase your self-confidence and reduce the symptoms associated with mild depression and anxiety. It can improve your sleep, which is often disrupted by stress, depression, and anxiety (see "Sleep It Off" on page 53), and give you a sense of command over your body and your life. You will most likely feel less stressed after you do your Yoga for Your Core or your Core+ routine because these workouts focus your attention on your breath instead of the daily stressors in your life.

EXERCISE: STRESS PREVENTER

Research shows that a daily dose of exercise can also change your brain to help you resist stress.

Scientists at Princeton University showed how this worked in laboratory rats. One group of rats was allowed to run, while the other group refrained from any form of exercise. Afterward, all of the rats were placed in a stressful situation by swimming in cold water. The findings? The scientists found that brain cells created from exercise in the running group appeared to be resistant to stress.[7]

And scientists at the University of Colorado Boulder found almost the same thing: Rats that had been allowed to run for several weeks before being given a stressful experience produced less brain chemicals associated with stress. Also, scientists the University of Houston injected rats with chemicals that create stress and found that the ones who had been allowed to exercise shrugged it off and behaved like normal, healthy rats. The couch-potato rats freaked out and hid.

So what does this mean for us? Basically, science is proving that the positive impacts of exercise prepares the cells within your brain to handle unexpected stress. Now, it's important to remember that these effects won't happen over-night—it can take a few weeks to get the full effect from your workouts. But

mat motivation
My Ultimate Attitude Challenge

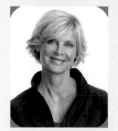

I know changing the way you think is easier said than done. But when I talk about the importance of having the right attitude if you want to trim your belly, I'm drawing on some pretty deep experience.

Back in my twenties, when I was diagnosed with terminal brain cancer, I was faced with a tough choice: Throw in the towel or fight like hell. You probably have a pretty good idea by now of which way I went.

To tell you the truth, I was furious—I mean really furious. I remember thinking, "Who the hell does this doctor think he is, telling me that I have 6 months to live?" Looking at him, I thought to myself: "I can run circles around him." I may have had a brain tumor, but I was an athlete and I wasn't about to let some MD who couldn't beat me in a 100-yard dash tell me I was going to die.

So here's what I did: I channeled my anger into fighting the cancer. And there was a lot of anger to channel. I had grown up really poor and was the first one in my family to go to college, then the first to go to law school. And the cancer diagnosis came during my last semester of law school. Imagine being so close to achieving your dream, then being told you're going to die.

Getting angry and channeling my rage saved my life. When I got out of the hospital, I took my training to a whole new level and actually became a professional triathlete. I was determined to show that not only had I survived, but I was thriving. In the years after, I became stronger and healthier than ever before.

There's no way that ever would have happened if I had the wrong attitude. Don't get me wrong, I'm not saying that every cancer patient can beat the disease with an attitude adjustment. Hopefully, you will never have to face this situation. But what I do know is that while we all struggle with fear and doubt, it's when you make up your mind to overcome any obstacle that your life really begins.

by the end of your Flat Belly Yoga! 4-Week Workout, you should start to notice the difference.

YOGA AND STRESS

Keep in mind, you're not just working out. You're doing the Flat Belly Yoga! Workout, and yoga has been proven to be *the best* exercise there is for stress relief. Scientists know that a brain chemical with the tongue-twisting name of gamma-aminobutyric acid—they call it GABA for short—is especially powerful at fighting depression and anxiety. And yoga is better than other forms of exercise at boosting GABA.

Researchers from Boston University School of Medicine have found that yoga may be superior to other forms of exercise in its positive effect on mood and anxiety. The findings are the first to demonstrate an association between yoga postures, increased GABA levels, and decreased anxiety.[8]

Scientists think it's because yoga poses are especially good at turning on specific nerves linked to the parasympathetic nervous system, which is responsible for helping you to relax.

SLEEP IT OFF

Not only will exercise help you if you're a stress case, it will also help you get some shut-eye. At Northwestern University, scientists took older women who had trouble sleeping and put them on a regular exercise program where they walked or used a stationary bike or treadmill four times a week.

Exercise improved the participants' self-reported sleep quality, elevating them from a diagnosis of "poor sleeper" to "good sleeper." They also reported fewer depressive symptoms, more vitality, and less daytime sleepiness.[9]

And other studies have shown that the amount of physical activity you do during the day is key to helping you sleep at night. The more active your body is during the day, the more likely you are to relax fully and fall asleep easily at night. With regular exercise like walking, your sleep quality also improves.

Exercise simply relaxes the body and calms the mind. It also helps reduce depression and anxiety—two common causes of sleeping disorders. Exercise sends signals to the body that more and deeper sleep at night is needed. It's important to note that improvement in sleep may not happen right away; it may not be apparent until a week or two after beginning an exercise program. But it will come.

Exercise also causes a significant rise in body temperature, followed by a compensatory drop a few hours later. The drop in body temperature, which persists for 2 to 4 hours after exercise, makes it easier to fall asleep and stay asleep because low body temperature coincides with low adrenaline. And when your adrenaline is at its lowest, you feel the most tired and therefore are able to sink into a deeper sleep.

Exercise, especially yoga, also eases the muscular tension that can build up in your body. One of the main reasons people can't get a good night's sleep is due to pain and stiffness. Yoga can help with both of these issues by promoting flexibility. It also sharpens the brain by increasing the amount of oxygen available.

You know by now that working out increases the body's production of endorphins. But did you know that endorphins create a sense of well-being and increase the body's resistance to pain, which help you sleep? Exercise also stimulates the release of epinephrine, a hormone that creates a sense of happiness and excitement and reduces boredom, worry, and tension.

Finally, exercise improves sleep because it is a physical stressor to the body. The brain compensates for physical stress by increasing deep sleep. Therefore, we sleep more deeply and soundly after exercise.

Taking all of this into consideration, it's also important to think about how our bodies fall asleep. Sleep is actually brought on by the release of chemicals in your body. These chemicals are a by-product of your body burning sugar for fuel during the day. The more sugar you burn (in other words, the more active you are), the more of these chemicals are released, aiding your sleeping habits.

Some people, though, find that exercise wakes them up. They have trouble sleeping if they exercise too late in the day. Try to exercise 20 to 30 minutes a day, about 5 to 6 hours before going to bed. Try to track your sleeping habits every day in your Flat Belly Yoga! Journal so that you know your best time to exercise.

Sleep and Fat

Scientists have known for years that not getting enough sleep increases levels of a hunger hormone and decreases levels of a hormone that makes you feel full. The effects may lead to overeating and weight gain. In the last few years, more and more research has been done on how lack of sleep hinders weight loss. In fact, a study from the *Annals of Internal Medicine* shows that cutting back on sleep by three hours a night while dieting can decrease weight lost as fat by as much as 55 percent.[10]

But here's some good news. According to Nathaniel F. Watson, MD, a neurologist and codirector of the University of Washington Medicine Sleep Center in Seattle, getting more sleep lessens the impact of your genes on your weight. So don't assume that because your family has a history of struggling with belly fat that you're doomed to the same fate. Simply getting a few more winks at night can help you lower your number on the scale.

And by giving you a good night's sleep, the Flat Belly Yoga! Workout offers one more way to help you say good-bye to your belly for good.

SUCCESS STORY

Shira Shimoni

Age: 40

Pounds lost:

3.5

in 32 days

All-over inches lost:

9

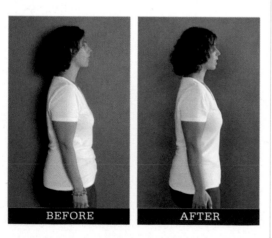

BEFORE | AFTER

" I was about to turn 40 and wanted to start the decade with a program that would flatten my belly once and for all," says Shira Shimoni. In the past, she used her birthdays as incentives to change her diet, but not necessarily her activity level. "In my thirties, I completely revamped my lifestyle and habits. I quit smoking and dropped 55 pounds, but it was all through dieting. As a result, my stomach and some other areas were a bit flabby and needed some focus."

As Shira knows, having a major event take place (whether it's getting married, having your high school reunion, or, in her case, turning 40) can make you reevaluate your current health and body image. It can propel you to stay committed to your current workout program, or even start a new one, by giving you that extra incentive to look good and feel great. And that's exactly what pushed Shira to give the Flat Belly Yoga! Workout a try. But shortly after beginning the program, she realized the one event that encouraged her to try a new plan would also be her first and biggest hurdle.

Shira's family and friends were flying in to partake in a 2-week celebration for her birthday. And dieting and exercise were not a part of that plan. So although she originally intended to follow the Flat Belly Diet! along with the Flat Belly Yoga! Workout, Shira found herself struggling to adhere to the diet during those 2 weeks. "I did better than I expected, but nonetheless I ate a lot of things I shouldn't have for my birthday," she laments. "The good news is that I did complete all of my workouts." In fact, one night while everyone else was celebrating her birthday, Shira did the Flat Belly Yoga! Workout with two of her visiting friends. And she even skipped some of her regular social events in order to prioritize her workouts. "It's really all about making the commitment to yourself and finding what works for you."

As she progressed further into the 4-Week Workout, the 40-year-old began to notice positive changes in her body. "My stomach was flatter after the first week," she says. "And as the weeks went by, I noticed more definition in my arms. Now my clothing fits better and my body is more defined. I feel a lot stronger and I look leaner." And these changes only reinforced her commitment to the program. "The workout was great and very accessible under any circumstances. I went out of town for a weekend and it was easy to keep up with my yoga workout and the Heart Walks. It was easy because it's a fun workout."

By the end of the program, Shira not only looked better, but she felt better, too. Working out on a regular basis kept her from thinking negatively about her body. If fact, Shira says that because the Flat Belly Yoga! Workout was such a positive experience, she plans to incorporate the program into her daily life in the future. "I will say that since I started the program, I no longer just glisten when I work out. I sweat—and I love it! This is just the beginning.

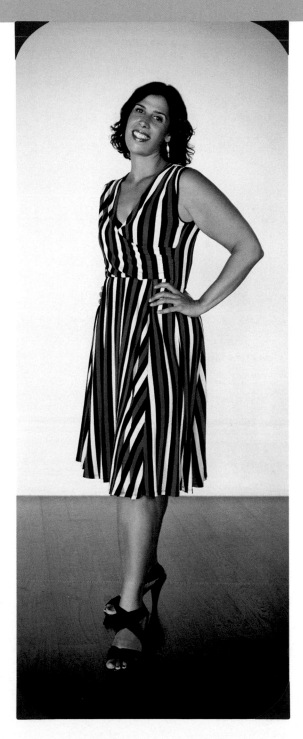

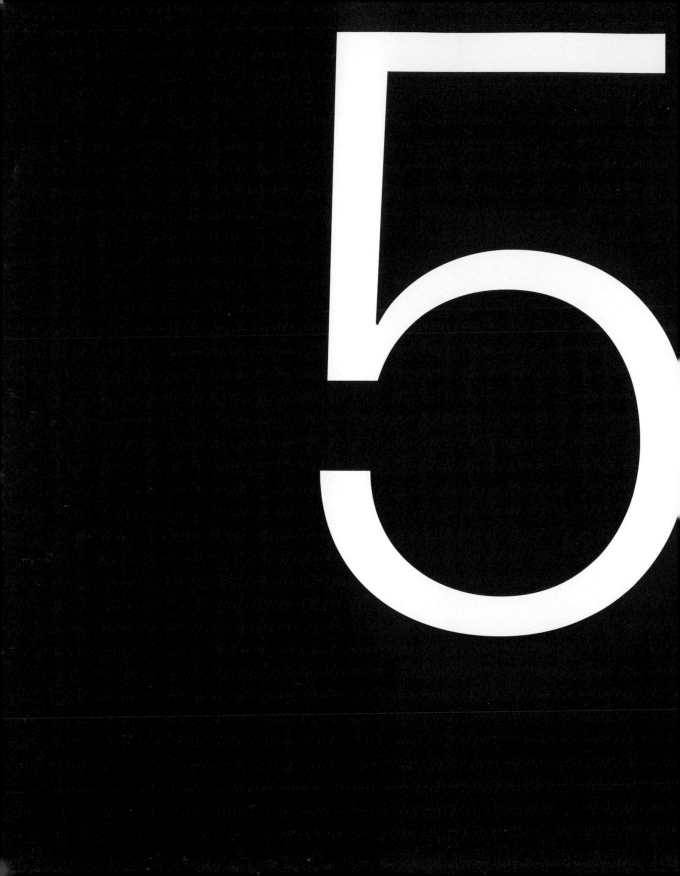

RULES OF ENGAGEMENT

The Flat Belly Yoga! Workout is designed to be safe, fun, and effective. But I still want you to check out these easy rules to ensure you're getting the best results from your workouts. Here we address common exercise best practices and get specific with special tips and pointers on how to safely complete your workout.

So be sure to read through this chapter before beginning your workout. It covers everything from what you should wear to making your workouts fun.

Start Small

When I say "start small," I mean don't overdo it. One of the most common mistakes people make when they are starting out is that they get excited about their new goals and push themselves too hard, too fast. It's good to be excited. Your intention to give yourself a flat belly is worth getting excited about. But if you push yourself too hard, you will feel sore the next day, and that will slow down your progress.

Remember, it's a marathon, not a sprint. That might not sound good to you, but what I mean is that you need to build your fitness base first. You should work out because you want to—because it makes you feel good all day. If you feel too sore and achy the next day, you won't want to keep working out. And we want to avoid that because it's more important to get into the habit of exercising. For starters, one of my goals is just to get you off the couch and onto the mat. My other goal is to make you feel so good about working out that you want to keep going.

But that's *my* goal. *Your* goal is to take it one a day at a time and make sure you feel good about your workout each and every day. The Flat Belly Yoga! Workout intensifies as it goes on. So you start with shorter walk times and yoga poses without weights, and then work up to longer walking times and Core+ Yoga with weights.

So as you bump it up, I want to make sure you listen to your body. I can't be there to do this for you. Sometimes we have a tendency to just push through and do what needs to be done. The problem, when we start exercising, is that approach can lead to injuries. And when you get hurt, your workouts go out the window. Not only will you have to take some days off, but you also won't want to start up again. And that's the opposite of what I want for you.

Instead, dial it back. Injuries can happen, but they happen most often when people get too tough on themselves and ignore what their bodies are telling them. I don't want you to ignore it if something hurts, especially when it comes to yoga. As incredible as yoga is for building your core and helping you get a flat belly, it must be done correctly.

MAKING REALISTIC PLANS

In order to meet your goal to start working out, we need to make sure your plans are realistic. So you need to set goals based on where your body *really* is right now. Tomorrow you'll find you can do a little bit more, and then a little bit more the next day. *Flat Belly Yoga!* is set up to take the guesswork out of your workout. All you need to do is follow the workout plan and not push yourself harder than instructed.

I know that after a week of doing the workout and listening to your body, you'll start to feel better about your abilities. Doing your Heart Walks and Core+ Yoga routines will begin to make you feel better and better. But I don't want you to jump to Week 4 because you are starting to feel good from working out. It's like following a recipe—you could change it, but it might not turn out the way you want it to. And the Flat Belly Yoga! Workout is a recipe for a flat belly, so let's stick to it!

On the other hand, maybe your body isn't feeling great today. Maybe traffic was bad and you sat for too long in the car. Maybe you slept funny last night and your neck feels tight. Or maybe you don't even know why it's happening, but things just aren't as easy as they should be. You're finding you can't quite do a movement or hold a pose that was easy for you to do yesterday or your calves are burning after only half of your Heart Walk.

If that's the case, *back it off.* It is normal for your body to go through ups and downs. If you imagine your progress as a graph, overall it's going to keep going up and up, but there will still be lots of peaks and valleys. It's okay if today you are in a valley. Don't try to force your way out of it.

ARE YOU HAVING FUN YET?

Here's a rule to live by: Have fun with your workouts. If you're not having fun, you probably won't continue to do it. Like I said in the beginning of this chapter, this book was designed to be safe, fun, and effective. I've made it safe and effective for you, but I need your help to make it fun.

Finding a workout buddy is a big help because being accountable to someone else helps you stay motivated. And, of course, it's fun to work out with a friend.

Are you reluctant to work out because you will miss time with your family or friends? Then enlist their help to make your Heart Walks more social. When your friends or family know that you are doing this workout plan to get and stay healthy, they will likely jump at the chance to help you stick to it. Plus, keeping up a conversation won't just make the minutes and miles go by—it will also give you a good gauge to make sure you aren't overdoing it or underdoing it!

According to researchers, exercising with a friend will make you feel better than working out alone. When we exercise, happiness hormones called

Mat Motivation
Meet Me at the Studio

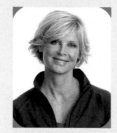

Want to hang out with me? Well, then, you better lace up your sneakers and head over to the studio. When it comes to working out, I'm all about joining a fitness community. In fact, I designed my business around this.

When I opened my first YAS Fitness Center, I wanted it to be the *Cheers* of workout studios. You might not remember the show *Cheers*, which was set in a bar in Boston and the theme was, "Where everyone knows your name." It's challenging to keep that feeling as you grow a company, but luckily I've been able to achieve it.

Now, I'm not saying to discard any friend who won't join you at a fitness center. But here's what I've found: Building my social life around my workouts is good for my body and for my emotional health. And even though my workout situation may be a little different from yours, I still have to find ways to motivate myself. And there's no better incentive than spending time with people you like.

I see this all the time at YAS. In fact, a lot of my students will tell their friends, "I'm going to YAS." That's different than saying, "I'm going to work out." It means they think of YAS Fitness Centers as a community—a meeting ground—not just an exercise facility.

Here's my advice for sustaining a workout routine: Find the thing that gets you going. Remember, it's more than exercise—there has to be an emotional attachment that keeps you engaged. And while you're at it, don't set false expectations. It's better to set realistic goals and achieve them. See you at the studio?

endorphins are released by the body, giving us a natural high and a feeling of elation, while also helping to reduce the feeling of pain. To find out if this hormone release is affected by working out in a group, a team of scientists from the University of Oxford measured endorphin production in a group of rowers, both when they exercised alone and when they trained together as a team.[1] Their results showed that sportsmen have a significantly higher tolerance to pain after exercising in a group than they do after exercising alone, suggesting that group workouts lead to a greater production of feel-good endorphins. And this could be a way to help humans bond in groups and improve social interactions.

So what if you can't seem to find someone to exercise with you? Lack of motivation can be a big obstacle to continuing your workouts, especially when you first start working out because you haven't developed the discipline yet. Well, that's why we start with the 4-Day Jump Start in Chapter 6 (see page 73). It gives you a chance to figure out what works for you. When it comes to walking, which will be your cardio component, there are a number of other ways to make it fun.

As you saw in Chapter 4, you can start by adding your favorite music. But it doesn't necessarily *have* to be music that you listen to while you walk. Music is a great motivator because your body naturally responds to it, but the important thing is not to be bored so that your walks are always a fun experience. One alternative to listening to music is checking out podcasts. There are hundreds and hundreds of them on every topic—news, science, health, entertainment, travel, philosophy, sports, cooking, you name it. And most of them are free. You can also listen to an audio book and get lost in a story (but not so lost that you stop paying attention to what's around you). You can even use your hands-free device and talk to a friend on the phone. As I mentioned earlier, talking to a friend is a great way to make sure you're not pushing yourself too hard or taking it too easy. You should be able to maintain a conversation, but just barely.

Regardless of how you customize your workouts to best suit your interests, don't forget the ultimate motivational tool: looking at yourself in the mirror and seeing a flat and toned belly!

Rules for Yoga

When you start any workout routine, you should take it slow. And with yoga, the slower you do the poses, the more muscles you are going to use. So for maximum benefits, slow it down! Here are some other rules to keep in mind:

Find the right place to do your yoga workouts. If you have a family or pets, it might be good to find a place that has some privacy (like the spare bedroom, if you have one). You want to make sure you stay focused. You don't want to be distracted. Any flat, open stretch of floor where you can shut the door and have some "me time" is perfect.

Know your limits and stay within them. Start with the basics. We begin your Flat Belly Yoga! Workout with Yoga for Your Core (part of the 4-Day Jump Start that starts on page 73). I've designed some core moves that will get you in touch with your soon-to-be flat belly. This is so you can get a feel for your form in the yoga poses before you add weights in the Core+ Yoga section. Yoga is all about moving slowly from one pose to the other. Going in and out of a pose in yoga is still part of the pose. It's not a time to take a little mini-break—you do not want to switch from one pose to the next without thinking about it. The transitions in between are very important, and the goal is to transition from pose to pose with as little excess movement as possible.

Keeping it smooth and slow not only gives you the best workout—it also protects you from injury by letting you feel where your limits are so you don't accidentally jerk past them. Swinging your weights, while it's easier for that split second, makes it more likely that a muscle or a joint will suddenly have more stress than it can handle.

If you start to feel like it's too hard to go slow and steady from one pose to the next, you can ease up. Remember that in this workout, the saying *no pain, no gain* does not apply. Yoga isn't supposed to hurt. If you feel any pain, stop. If you find a pose is too hard to hold, try holding it for a shorter time.

Don't skip the warm-up. There is a reason for it: Warming up helps you avoid getting hurt.

Warming up prior to any physical activity has a number of benefits. But its main purpose is to prepare the body and mind for more strenuous activity. One of the ways it achieves this is by increasing the body's core temperature and muscle temperature. The increase in muscle temperature helps make your muscles loose, supple, and pliable.

An effective warm-up also has the effect of increasing both your heart rate and your respiratory rate. This increases blood flow, which in turn aids in the delivery of oxygen and nutrients to the working muscles. All of this helps to prepare the muscles, tendons, and joints for more strenuous activity.[2]

Keep this in mind as you get stronger. Don't hurry through the warm-up because it seems too easy. It is supposed to be easy. It's getting your body ready for your workout.

Be aware of your body. Yoga is all about body awareness. No other workout has you focus on one side of your body independently from the other. In a lot of other workouts, your body would just compensate, meaning your stronger side

What Should I Wear?

I get asked this question all the time: "Kimberly, what should I wear to do yoga?" I know there are a lot of very expensive yoga clothing companies. But honestly, you don't need to wear anything special. Think about what you would wear to the gym. Anything you can move around in comfortably is fine.

When it comes to picking out your walking shoes, find a store that has staff who know what they are doing. You should have them measure your feet, even if you think you know your size. Sometimes our sizes change over the years. The rule of thumb is that you want a thumb's distance from your toe to the top of your sneaker.

Don't buy shoes based on how they look or because you like the style or saw a celebrity wearing them. Pick the right shoe for your foot type. You also want to change your sneakers every 300 to 500 miles. If you can't remember how long you've had your sneakers, you might want to start your Flat Belly Yoga! Workout with a new pair. Then you can leave those new shoes by the door to remind yourself to take your Heart Walk each day.

would take up the slack for your weaker side. Unfortunately, in that scenario, your body will never be balanced—your strong side will always remain stronger.

Luckily for us, the Flat Belly Yoga! Workout is all about balance. I want you to notice the imbalances between the sides of your body—which side is stronger, which side is more flexible—and write down what you notice in your journal (see Chapter 9 on page 177).

Focus on your breath. Before you even start to feel pain or soreness in your body, your breath can tell you if you're pushing yourself too hard. It is the early warning system for the rest of your body. You should be able to take deep, full breaths throughout your workout. If you can't—and if you notice that your breath has become labored or you can't manage to pull in a full breath—then something is wrong. Either you have pushed yourself too hard overall and have become too tired, or you are pushing yourself too hard in a particular pose, past where your body is ready to go.

Rarely does this happen in yoga, unless you're taking a rigorous Power Yoga class, or you're in a Bikram Hot Yoga class where the temperature in the room is heated to 105 degrees Fahrenheit. But be mindful of this anyway.

And remember, just because your body went there yesterday doesn't mean it is ready to go there again today. Pay attention to what your body is telling you: It knows more than you give it credit for. Keep in mind that focusing on your breath and your body is part of what makes yoga such a great stress buster. Don't cheat yourself out of that!

Rules for Walking

When it comes to doing your Heart Walks, the number one rule is to be safe. There are several ways to make them safe.

Warm up first. Just as with your yoga workouts, your warm-ups are included in your Heart Walk program. Start slow and then increase the intensity of your walk. Make sure you cool down after your walk, too.

Walk in a familiar area. Think of places like your neighborhood, or places not too far from where you work. Make sure you're familiar with the surrounding areas as well.

Bring a light. If you are buying new shoes, buy ones that have reflective tape on them. If you have decided to walk at night, then bring a flashlight with you. Whether you are walking during the day or at night you might want to wear brightly colored clothes so people can see you.

Don't carry a purse. Just put your keys and cell phone in your pocket. (You want to make sure whatever you are wearing has pockets.) I love listening to music when I walk, but you need to keep the volume at a level where you can hear someone coming up behind you.

Using Weights

Set it down. Is this the first time you've used weights? If so, remember that you can always put your weights down and do the workout without them if it becomes too difficult.

Use proper form. To get the best results from your Core+ Yoga Workout, you need to make sure you're holding each pose correctly. In addition to getting the most out of your workout, you're also less likely to hurt yourself. So before adding weights to your routine, take a look at the photos beginning on page 108 to learn how to use proper form while incorporating weights into your yoga routine. And don't forget: It's also important to maintain proper form when you are picking up and putting down weights to avoid injury.

Don't swing your weights. It's important to remember to use your muscles, not momentum, to move your weights. If you find that you can't do the movements for your Core+ poses without swinging your weights around, I would suggest trying lighter weights (see Chapter 2 on page 17 for more details).

Well-Watered Exerciser

With the exception of oxygen, water is actually the most important thing your body needs. The more you exercise, the more important it is to drink the right amount of water. Make sure to drink before, during, and after your workouts to prevent dehydration. However, drinking too much water at the wrong time can also hinder performance.

So how do you know how much you need to drink and when to drink it? Obviously, people differ greatly in body size, how much they sweat, the type and amount of exercise they do, and the climate in which they exercise. So with all these factors it's hard to make a one-size-fits-all recommendation on drinking water. But here are some general guidelines:

If your typical exercise session is around 60 minutes or less and doesn't involve vigorous activity outdoors in hot, humid weather, you probably don't need to interrupt your exercise session for a drink. A healthy, average-sized person can produce as much as 32 ounces of sweat during an hour of moderate to vigorous indoor exercise. That may feel and look like a lot of sweating, but it shouldn't be enough to cause problems unless you've been seriously shortchanging yourself on fluid intake prior to starting your exercise. You can tell whether that's a potential problem by checking your urine color before exercise. If it's dark yellow with a strong urine smell, it's a good idea to have a cup or two of water 30 to 60 minutes before you start exercising. If it's clear to light yellow, it should be fine to just rehydrate gradually after your exercise session without worrying about stopping to drink in the middle of it.

According to the American College of Sports Medicine, dehydration is likely to start affecting exercise performance when sweating causes you to lose 2 percent or more of your normal (hydrated) body weight.[3] That's more than 51 ounces, or a little over 3 pounds, for an average person of 160 pounds. At this level of mild dehydration, you'll probably be a little thirsty (though many people don't experience thirst until they're already dehydrated), and you may start to feel as if you have to work significantly harder to maintain your performance level. As dehydration gets progressively more severe, you may start to feel lightheaded, uncoordinated, or have muscle cramps. To avoid these symptoms, make sure to check your hydration before and after your workouts. It'll also give you the energy you need to successfully complete the workout at hand.

 If you are walking, jogging, or doing yoga outside, make sure the area is safe or bring a friend with you.

Get a Gauge

Start the Flat Belly Yoga! program with your own weigh-in before you begin the Jump Start in the following chapter. Also take your measurements and write those below as well. You will be amazed when you look back to see how far you have come in just 32 days!

Start Date	
WEIGHT:	WAIST: (The most important number!)
CHEST:	HIPS:
LEFT BICEP:	RIGHT BICEP:
LEFT THIGH:	RIGHT THIGH:

A FLAT BELLY YOGA
SUCCESS STORY

Nathalie Roque

Age: 32

Pounds lost:
3
in 32 days

All-over inches lost:
13

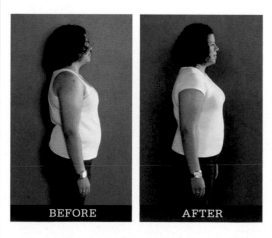

BEFORE   AFTER

" I could never find a great balance between work, health, and my personal life. I would always make excuses as to why I couldn't take the time to exercise," admits Nathalie Roque, who works in advertising. In the past, Nathalie always chose to spend extra time at the office instead of at the gym because she felt work was more important. And because her job requires long hours of sitting, she was getting little to no exercise throughout the day.

Because she had such a difficult time even knowing when to leave her office, Nathalie knew she needed a plan that would offer structure and balance—two things she'd always wanted, but didn't know how to achieve. So when the opportunity to try the Flat Belly Yoga! Workout came along, Nathalie thought this could finally be the chance to learn how to incorporate exercise into her daily life.

She also knew she needed to start at a slower pace in order to succeed in the program. "In the past, I tried to be perfect, and I learned there is no such thing as being perfect," she states. "I accepted the possibility that I might not stick to this 100 percent, and that was okay—just as long as I did not let it completely slip."

So to ensure she would stick to her workouts on busy days, the 32-year-old had to create a realistic plan that would work every day—regardless of what was happening in the office. And for Nathalie, that meant scheduling daily workout appointments in her calendar—something she had never done before. "I would look at my work schedule and what I had going on in my life, find time in the morning or afternoon to work out, and made it my mission to make it happen," she says. "I not only formatted my fancy new iPhone, but also my work calendar to make sure at least 30 minutes to an hour out of the day was dedicated to leaving my desk and going for a walk."

She also made sure to include her yoga workouts when she knew she would have some spare time—first thing in the morning. "I managed to wake up early to do the yoga-with-weights routine in the morning as a precaution. I knew that if my day ever got hectic, it was okay, because I had already started out a great day by doing my workout."

And as a bonus, Nathalie also learned how to balance her diet. At her office, vendors would bring in cupcakes and host happy hours, so she was constantly exposed to sugary foods. Instead of joining her coworkers for midday snacks, Nathalie would go on her Heart Walk. "I learned how to say no and cut back on sweets and food that was not healthy."

By the end of the 32-day program, Nathalie lost an astonishing 6 inches from her belly! "This is the first time I have seen an improvement," she exclaims. "In the beginning, there were times I felt like quitting, but I kept visualizing that at the end, this would be the first program I started and finished—without cheating or quitting. I am so thankful to Kimberly, my family, and, really, myself for cheering me on and telling me that I could do it. 99

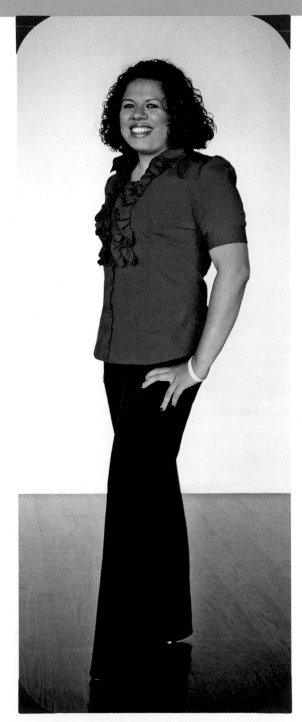

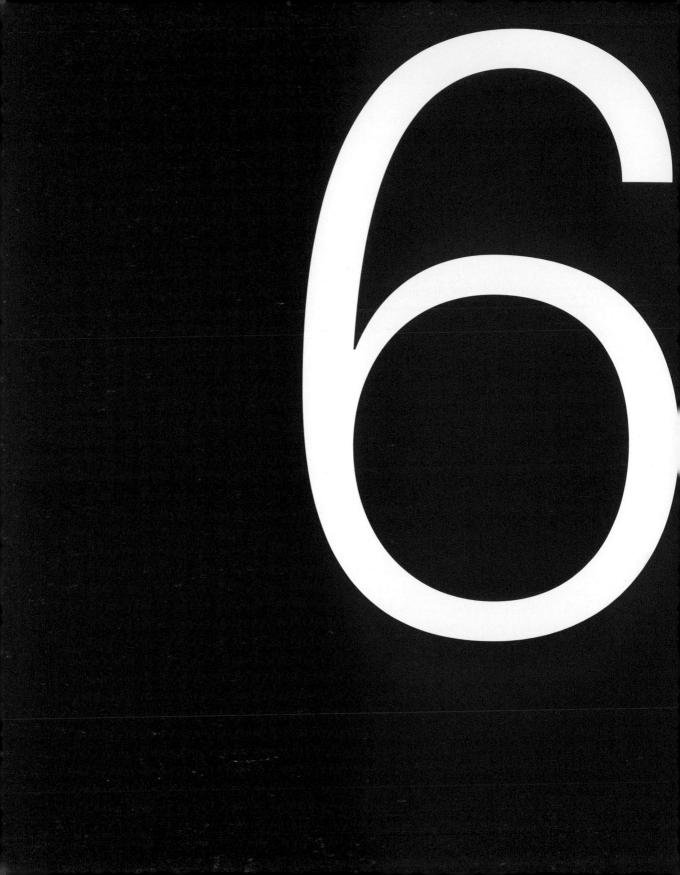

JUMP-START YOUR WORKOUT!

It's time to begin your Flat Belly Yoga! 4-Day Jump Start. If you're a little skittish about exercise, the Jump Start is a perfect way to get you warmed up to the idea of a daily exercise routine. *This is something you can do!*

The Jump Start combines low-intensity yoga with Heart Walk cardio sessions to get you off the couch and moving around. The yoga portion of the Jump Start, also known as Yoga for Your Core, starts with just a few simple, straightforward moves that happen to be some of my favorite easy stretches.

Once you finish the first 4 days, you'll begin the 4-Week Workout, a 28-day exercise plan that combines Core+ Yoga (designed specifically to strengthen your core) with Heart Walks that will raise your heart rate and burn off belly fat.

If you already work out or do yoga, you might be tempted to skip the Jump Start and plunge right into the 4-Week Workout. But I'm going to advise you not to do that: It's important to get used to the Yoga for Your Core sequence before adding weights in order to prevent injury. And there's no hurry. It will put you ahead in the long term.

Maybe you're a bit of a couch potato. Maybe you never meant to be this way, but because of our addiction to e-mail and social media, you have fallen into a sedentary lifestyle. Maybe you have an aversion to exercise, or you've been burned one too many times by exercise programs that promised you unattainable results and set you up for failure.

If any of these scenarios sound familiar, then the 4-Day Jump Start was made for you. It will reintroduce you to a healthy, active exercise routine that will set the

The Flat Belly Diet!

Are you doing this workout program in conjunction with the Flat Belly Diet!? This book was designed so that you can easily incorporate the Flat Belly Diet! meal plan for even better results. Both plans begin with a 4-Day Jump Start—referred to as the 4-Day Anti-Bloat Jump Start in the *Flat Belly Diet!* (see Chapter 10 on page 205 for a summary of the meal plan).

Created to shrink your belly by conquering bloat, the 4-Day Anti-Bloat Jump Start will place you on a restricted-calorie diet of 1,200 calories per day. It's especially important that you not start the 4-Week Workout (see page 103) at the same time you're doing the 4-Day Anti-Bloat Jump Start. If you're on a calorie-restricted diet, you're going to want to take it a little easier, and you should. But the low-intensity exercise of the Flat Belly Yoga! Jump Start fits perfectly with the first 4 days of the diet—they were designed to be done at the same time to ease you into the program.

stage for your success. I created the Jump Start to introduce you to the yoga poses essential to the Flat Belly Yoga! Workout. You'll master these poses in the next 4 days, which will give you the confidence to stick with the program and get back on track to a healthier and happier you—no matter what shape you're in today.

Start at the Beginning

Regardless of your diet plans and exercise level (whether you're an avid exerciser or a couch potato), I recommend you start here, at the beginning. There's no reason to push too hard too soon—I'd much rather that you build up to the 4-Week Workout with the Jump Start, and research agrees with me. When the Centers for Disease Control (CDC) looked at women in military basic training, they found clear evidence that the choice of workout program should be in line with a woman's level of physical fitness. And beginning an exercise routine that's too difficult can increase your risk for injury by as much as 3.5 times.[1] So, remember to take it slow. And don't worry if it feels slow now because we're going to ramp it up in just 4 days!

Making Time for You!

To start the Flat Belly Yoga! Workout, you need to get in the habit of *taking care of yourself first*—and this can be hard. Women, in particular, receive negative reinforcement for putting ourselves first, while we get positive reinforcement for putting our families, friends, and colleagues before ourselves. We need to change that, and we need to change it every day.

It's important to try extra hard to not just exercise here and there for a month. There's a reason I want you to put yourself first and exercise every day (with one day of rest each week in the upcoming 4-Week Workout) for a whole month. And it's not because after that month, you'll be perfectly healthy for the rest of your life. If you've exercised before, you know better than that!

If you do this every day—especially when you're just starting out—you can turn daily exercise into a habit. Wouldn't it be great to have yoga as your habit, instead of smoking, biting your nails, or looking at Facebook? By committing to the first month of this new habit and repeating that commitment to yourself every day, you're going to make exercise an automatic part of your life.

Flat Belly Yoga! contains exercises that, if you keep doing them, will keep you healthy for the rest of your life. Right now, your number one reason to do yoga every day is probably to flatten your belly. But you'll start to see other life-changing benefits as well, such as stress reduction and time for reflection.

Ask yourself: How will your life change after you create the habit of doing yoga every day? How great would it be to develop the habit of putting yourself first?

OFF THE COUCH, ONTO THE MAT

Here's the good news: You've already made that first step toward putting yourself first. You picked up a book called *Flat Belly Yoga!*, so I'm willing to bet that either a) you want to try yoga, or b) you've tried it in the past, but maybe something about it wasn't quite right for you. Either way—whether it wasn't your thing or you just haven't gotten around to trying it—now you're ready to give it a chance.

Maybe you never thought that yoga was for you—maybe it sounded a little too "woo woo." (I talk about that in my previous book, *The No OM Zone*.) But if nothing else has worked to get rid of that undesirable belly fat, why not give yoga a chance?

After all, research shows that yoga is one of the best exercises to flatten, strengthen, and tone your belly. And one study in particular proved that practicing yoga regularly can significantly decrease weight, body fat percentage, waist circumference, and visceral fat (the dangerous fat surrounding your organs) in postmenopausal women. Furthermore, this same study showed that practicing yoga can even reduce your blood sugar levels and your blood pressure.[2]

So why should you start a yoga routine? The benefits are simply too good to pass up. And all you need to do to get started is get off of the couch and onto the mat. (Could that sound any easier?) I'm going to get you moving with some basic yoga poses that will ease you into the more intermediate poses of the 4-Week Workout.

HEART HEALTH

I'm also going to get you out the door and around your neighborhood. You're going to go for a Heart Walk every day. Every exercise program needs an element of cardio because part of getting and keeping you healthy is getting your heart rate up. Why is this so important? According to the CDC, cardiovascular disease is the leading cause of death among women. Take a look at some facts:

- In 2008, one in four women died from heart disease. As the number one killer of women, it often strikes at younger ages than most people realize, with middle-aged women especially at risk.[3]

- In 2008, more women died from heart disease than from every type of cancer combined (415,969 died from heart disease versus 270,210 women who died of cancer).[4]

- Cardiovascular disease is currently the third leading cause of disability among women, followed by arthritis and spine or back problems.[5]

The most common cause of heart disease is narrowing or blockage of the coronary arteries, the blood vessels that supply blood to the heart itself. This is called coronary artery disease and happens slowly over time. It's the major cause of all heart attacks, and prevention is key: Two-thirds of women who have a heart attack fail to make a full recovery. The good news is that anyone can take the steps to prevent this disease by practicing healthy lifestyle habits.[6]

Does that all sound a little heavier than what you expected to hear? I don't want you to follow the plan I've created in *Flat Belly Yoga!* because you're scared of death, disease, and disability. It's more important to me for you to feel empowered to take control of your health, and for you to enjoy exercise for how it makes you feel and look. But I also want you to be proud that you're taking care of *you*.

Weigh In

Before you start the 4-Day Jump Start, you might want to get naked and look at yourself in a full-length mirror. Sometimes we look better with clothes on, so this will help you get a gauge on your belly. Don't beat yourself up—just remind yourself of what you want to accomplish.

Next, hop on your scale and weigh yourself before we take this journey together. I weigh myself every day. By observing your weight as a matter of routine, it changes your weight from a problem you don't want to face into a daily piece of information, like the temperature or the date on the calendar. Think about it: When you have gotten to the point where you are 15 or more pounds too heavy, how did that happen? Was it because you stopped wanting to know, because you were afraid of the answer?

If you do weigh yourself every day, weight gain is less likely to sneak up on you without you knowing about it. You still might gain weight, but you will be aware of it happening. And it's more likely that by knowing what's going on, you'll make the changes to your routine, activity level, and diet to help you take control. Research clearly shows that people who weigh themselves on a daily basis lose more weight in the long run.

Researchers at the University of Minnesota and the Minneapolis Heart Institute Foundation found that there is a strong relationship between weekly weight checks and maintaining your weight loss. And if you choose to weight yourself daily, you're even more likely to maintain your weight loss over a long period of time. In fact, the study found that people who weighed themselves every day lost between 18 to 27 pounds more than those who chose not to weight themselves regularly.[7]

This research demonstrates just how strong the relationship is between regular weight checks and maintaining your weight loss. Even if you don't like what the scale has to say right now, that's going to change once you're on this program. So I'm going to strongly suggest that you start your Flat Belly Yoga! Workout with a weigh-in, and do one every day throughout the plan.

Where's the Time?

I know that when you first start this program, it might be hard to make the time to add both yoga and walking into your daily routine. At first, feel free to break up your walks into smaller increments. Let's say your goal is to do your Heart Walk for 30 minutes. Maybe it's easier for you to go for a 15-minute walk twice a day, or a 10-minute walk three times a day. You can take a break from your computer or TV and walk around the block. In Chapter 8 on page 163, I'll give you a number of tips to help you figure out how to find the time. No excuses! There is more time in your day than you realize—and if you make it, the rewards will be even bigger than you think.

I have always been active and chose to make my whole life about fitness. I went from trying to help myself get fit to helping others accomplish their fitness goals. Today, I'm a national fitness expert. I spend my whole life helping people just like you get healthy and lose weight. And I love my job!

Now, I don't want you to get the wrong idea from this story. Let's get one thing straight: You don't have to quit your job and become a fitness pro in order to find time to work out. As a fitness professional, the last thing I want to do is set your expectations too high. Instead, I want to help you find the right way to incorporate the workout that's right for you into your daily life. I'm assuming you're not a yoga pro, so let's begin with some basics.

Most of the yoga poses you will be doing in the Yoga for Your Core Routine will be incorporated in the 4-Week Workout. So now I want you to use the 4-Day Jump Start to build your foundation and establish a routine.

You're going to use your Flat Belly Yoga! Journal (see Chapter 9 on page 177) to help you figure out what time of day you most enjoy working out. It's important to know what works for you: If the Flat Belly Yoga! Workout gives you energy—and it might—then you will probably want to incorporate it into your morning routine to start out your day. You may choose to include it in your afternoon routine to give you the burst of energy you need after the lunchtime slump. Or maybe you're the kind of person who finds that exercise is just what you need to relax after a long day. In that case, try scheduling your workouts at night.

Remember that you'll also need to make time for a short walk (a Heart Walk) every day. There are several intensity levels of Heart Walks, but for your first four days, I just want to get you out of the house. (I recommend walking, but you can do any form of cardio that interests you—cycling, swimming, or jogging—as long as you're moving.)

Use your Flat Belly Yoga! Journal to gauge how you feel when you walk. Write down your time and distances walked. Keeping a daily journal allows you to track your progress, and seeing all those miles add up, one after another, is a powerful tool to keep you motivated! (See Chapter 9 for more details on how to start your journal.)

Are you ready to start?

Beginning the Jump Start

As you start the Flat Belly Yoga! Workout, keep in mind what I said about getting used to making exercise a permanent part of your lifestyle. It's worth repeating: You need to get in the habit of taking care of yourself first.

There will always be an excuse for why you don't have time to work out. Since the day you were born, no day ended the way you expected it to. Appointments get moved around; someone needs to be picked up. There's always something happening that you can use to justify stealing time from your workouts—and yourself. If an excuse comes up—and one will, probably every single day—write it in your Flat Belly Yoga! Journal. Then go ahead and do your workout anyway. You deserve it!

HEART WALKS

There are two types of walking workouts featured in the Flat Belly Yoga! Workout. If you want to lose belly fat, your walks need to be real workouts, which means we need to get your heart rate up.

Your aerobic program will include both steady pace and interval walks. The first type of walking is called Fat Blast. That's a fast-paced walk, meaning it's not leisurely. You will increase the distance you walk every week. You will find that as you become fitter and the program goes on, your muscles will get stronger and you will naturally walk faster. When you walk faster, you will lose more weight. Exciting, right? The best part is that as the weeks go on, this will all happen without the workout feeling any harder. It will happen because you're getting in shape.

The second type of walk is called Calorie Torch. This is an interval walk, meaning it shifts back and forth between a fast-paced walk and a series of high-intensity "bursts" in which you will be walking at a brisk pace. You'll start with a steady, fast-paced walk, and then you'll shift gears by moving into what I call a pick-me-up pace, which is your high-intensity pace. (When I lived in Houston, I used to run with my golden retriever, Weatherby, on a 3-mile dirt loop around Memorial Park. My coach at the time would run out of patience pretty quickly if I ever slowed down. "Fowler, pick it up!" he'd say. That's why the Heart Walks include pick-me-ups.)

Think of it this way: You're walking down the street at your steady, fast pace, and up ahead, you see a friend of yours down the street. And it's a friend you actually want to see. They're already walking at their own steady, fast pace (maybe they're even doing a Fat Blast), and you want to catch up with them. So you pick up your pace.

Remember, the pick-me-up pace is supposed to be high intensity to *you*, not to me or your cousin Ralph. Whether you're a triathlete or a couch potato, this workout is about pushing yourself out of your comfort zone. Walking at this level of intensity can burn 25 to 75 percent more calories than working out at a lower level.

The Calorie Torch incorporates intervals because it's unhealthy to maintain an extremely high level of intensity for the entire workout, unless you're a professional athlete. In that case, it should be a piece of cake!

Form Check—Head to Toe

To get the most out of your Heart Walks and to keep them injury free, let's focus on your form:

- Start at the top: Check your head! Keep your head and neck in line with your shoulders. Don't strain your neck by looking down. Keep your neck straight by looking a few feet in front of you. And remember that your chin should be parallel to the ground.

- Try to keep your shoulders back, and drop your shoulder blades down your back. This will help your arms move/swing freely.

- Make sure you keep your arms close to your body. Your elbows should be at a 90-degree angle so that your arms swing straight back and forth.

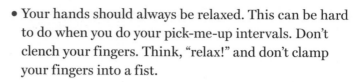

- Your hands should always be relaxed. This can be hard to do when you do your pick-me-up intervals. Don't clench your fingers. Think, "relax!" and don't clamp your fingers into a fist.

- Your foot strike is very important. Focus on your heel hitting the ground first. Then roll forward toward your toes. As one foot is rolling toward your toes, the other foot should be hitting the ground heel first.

- And remember: The Flat Belly Yoga! Workout is all about your core, so focus on your abs when you are walking by standing up straight. When it comes to your legs, move from your hips instead of your knees. (When you use your hip flexors to move your leg forward, the leg straightens and you will land on your heel, which is proper walking form.)

It really isn't that complicated, but it's similar to what your coach would tell you to do if you were running. So right now, I'm your walking coach!

PLAY IT SAFE Get a good pair of walking or running shoes. It really does make a difference. It's not fun walking in tight-fitting shoes.

Move with a Purpose

When you hear about cardio, you often hear that running or indoor cycling is the best form. In fact, walking, if done correctly, scores just as high when it comes to weight loss. It's also a lot easier on your joints. But when it comes to walking, you really need to get moving. You can't do a lazy walk and expect to lose weight.

So when you are walking, I want you to move with a purpose. And what's the purpose? *To lose your belly fat!* I know it's hard to know how hard you should be walking. Here's an easy trick you can use to gauge whether you're walking fast enough: Can you sing while you're walking? If so, you need to bump it up!

mat motivation

My Jump Start: How I Began a Career in Fitness

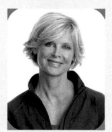 I know it's not easy to make a major change in your life, whether it's getting in shape or switching careers. But I'm here to tell you that it can be done. And I think an example from my own life might inspire you.

My background is basically a 180 from what I am doing now. I doubt you'll find another yoga expert with a similar history. I was the first person in my family to go to college, let alone law school. I put myself through school by working several jobs. I became a lawyer and was a litigator for 18 years. After that, I took on the task of becoming the chief operating officer for a $200-million vitamin company (sort of my first step into the health and wellness business.)

Having always been interested in fitness, I was a professional triathlete. I was also a bit of a daredevil. One day while I was out free climbing (climbing without ropes) near Las Vegas, I slipped on a patch of ice and fell about 30 feet. I impaled myself on a stump and my ribs went through my internal organs. I punctured my kidney in six places and popped my lung. Then I somehow had to climb back down the mountain.

I will not bore you with more details, but this was a game changer for me, as it put me in the hospital for about 6 months and I lost my job. I had a lot of time to think. So I kept asking myself, "What do you want to do with your life?"

This was a tragedy, but it was also an opportunity. I had always *loved* fitness. It had been a part of my life for as long as I could remember. At the time, my two favorite things to do were yoga and Spinning. I would take a yoga class, then drive across town and take a Spinning class and get so frustrated because no one had put the two together. Then one morning, while I was in the shower I had my *aha!* moment. Why couldn't I do it? And that's how YAS was born. I was the first person to put the two together. At the time, everyone thought I was crazy, but now they call me the "Godmother of Yoga Hybrids."

The lesson of this story is that you can make dramatic changes in your life. All it takes is the will to do it, a good plan, and persistence. I guarantee that if you apply this formula to getting a flat belly, soon you'll be sharing your own success story with others. So let's get moving!

YOGA

There's no putting it off—it's now time to start your yoga practice. Before I walk you through the Yoga for Your Core Routine step-by-step, let's first do a basic form check.

Starting with your head, let's stay focused. When you are doing your Heart Walk, you can think of anything you want. In yoga, not so much. As we saw in Chapter 1, one of the many things that makes yoga different from just stretching is the importance you place on how you breathe. Paying attention to breath work will help you always engage your core. And that's the most important element of the Flat Belly Yoga! Workout. It's the key to getting you the flat belly of your dreams.

Please read all the way through the Yoga for Your Core Routine before you try it. Looking at the photos as you go will help you understand and remember the poses and movements, so that when you start your workout, you can just follow the summary on page 86.

The Flat Belly Yoga! Jump Start

It doesn't matter in which order you do your workouts, whether you do your Heart Walk or Yoga for Your Core first. Just make sure you get them done. The first 4 days you should just plan on jump-starting your body and mind to get moving. Decide on your schedule. Write down your thoughts, how you feel, and what's stopping you from working out, if anything. It's good to start your workout by reminding yourself of your intention, or your motivation, for doing the Flat Belly Yoga! Workout. Write your intention in your Flat Belly Yoga! Journal (see Chapter 9). I've also included music playlists (see page 99) to accompany the Yoga for Your Core and Heart Walk routines. I know that during the first 4 days, you might need some extra motivation. I don't want to leave anything to chance. You should be all ready to go! I hope you're excited to get started. I know I'm excited for you!

As we move into the Flat Belly Yoga! 4-Week Workout, we will be adding a little more intensity with the Core+ Yoga routines.

Flat Belly Yoga! Jump Start Workout

	Day 1	**Day 2**	**Day 3**	**Day 4**
Heart Walk	**Fat Blast Walk** 20 minutes • 3-minute warm-up • 15-minute fast pace • 2-minute cooldown	**Calorie Torch Walk** 15 minutes • 3-minute warm-up • 10-minute fast pace with three 1-minute pick-me-ups • 2-minute cooldown	**Fat Blast Walk** 20 minutes • 3-minute warm-up • 15-minute fast pace • 2-minute cooldown	**Calorie Torch Walk** 15 minutes • 3-minute warm-up • 10-minute fast pace with three 1-minute pick-me-ups • 2-minute cooldown
Yoga Routine	**Yoga for Your Core** 15 minutes	**Yoga for Your Core** 15 minutes	**Yoga for Your Core** 15 minutes	**Yoga for Your Core** 15 minutes

Yoga for Your Core Routine

Pull out your yoga mat if you have one. If you don't, no problem—you can do your workout on a rug. Just make sure the rug is secured so it doesn't slip.

If you have kids, other family members, or pets, try to find an area where they won't be interrupting you during your yoga practice. You should also keep a glass of water and a towel nearby for convenience.

❶ Warm-Up/Breath Work
p. 88

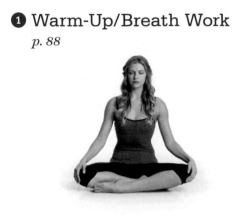

❹ Chair Pose
p. 91

❺ Warrior 1
p. 92

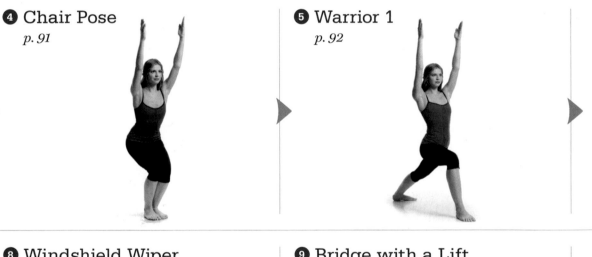

❽ Windshield Wiper
p. 96

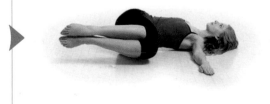

❾ Bridge with a Lift
p. 97

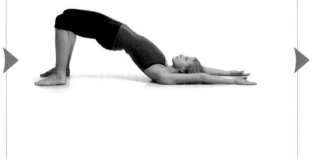

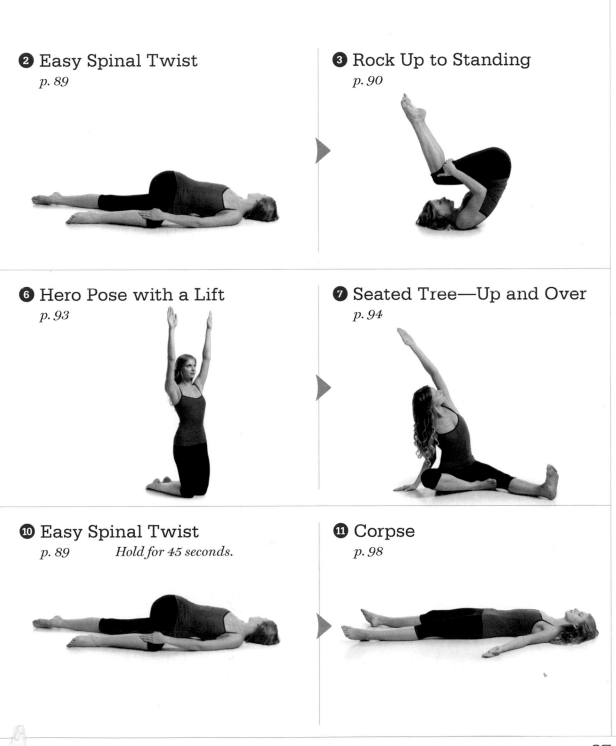

② Easy Spinal Twist
p. 89

③ Rock Up to Standing
p. 90

⑥ Hero Pose with a Lift
p. 93

⑦ Seated Tree—Up and Over
p. 94

⑩ Easy Spinal Twist
p. 89　　*Hold for 45 seconds.*

⑪ Corpse
p. 98

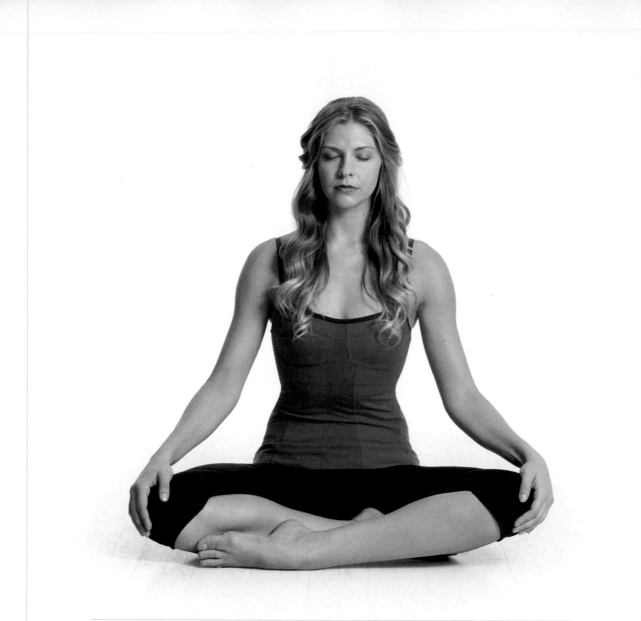

Warm-Up/Breath Work

Come to the floor for some breath work—it's a good way to start your Flat Belly Yoga! Jump Start Workout.

Sit in a cross-legged position, using your core to keep your back straight. Close your eyes and take a deep breath. Breathe in through your nose and out through your mouth. Let's do this 3 times. Take a deep breath in and see if you can hold it for a few seconds. Then let it go. Repeat this one more time.

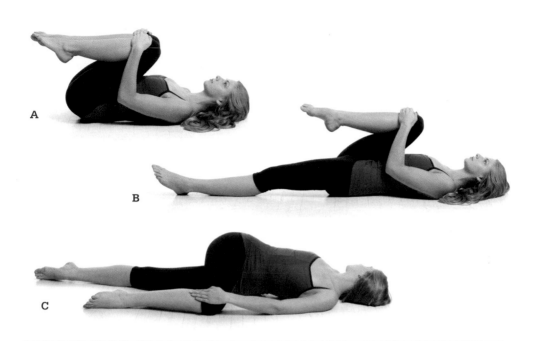

A

B

C

Easy Spinal Twist

A Bring your knees together and roll down onto your back. Hug your knees into your chest and gently rock side to side, massaging your lower back. **B** Keep your right knee into your chest and move your left leg straight out on the floor.
C Take a deep breath in. On your exhale, bring your right knee across your body toward the left side of the room while keeping your shoulder blades on the floor. Then bring your right arm straight out from your shoulder and look to the right.

Hold the stretch for 30 seconds, then switch sides. To do this, both knees should come back into your chest. This time your left knee stays in and your right leg goes straight onto the floor. Bring your left knee toward the right side of the room with your left arm straight out from your shoulder. Look out over your left shoulder. Take a second to notice if there was a difference between one side and the other. Hold for 30 seconds, then bring both knees to your chest.

mat matters

Don't try to force your knee down with your hand. This will lift your shoulder blade off the floor.

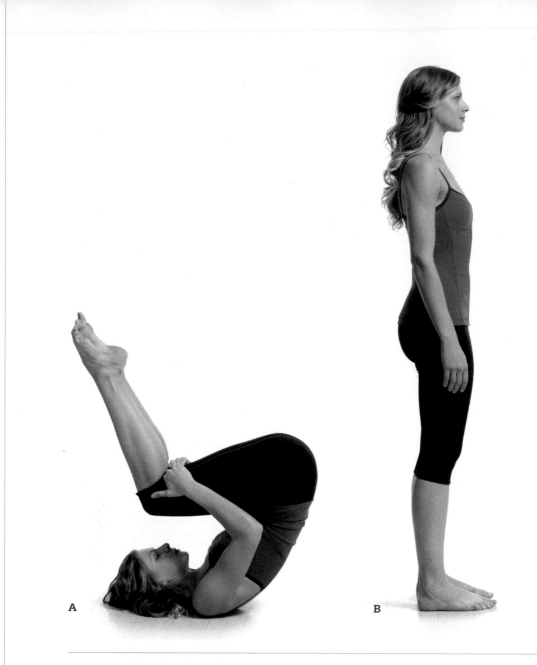

A   B

Rock Up to Standing

Ⓐ Lying on your back with both knees at your chest, rock back and forth from your shoulders to your hips. Ⓑ Once you get up the momentum, rock up onto your feet and stand up. This takes a lot of core strength, so you can make it easier by using your hands to push yourself up.

Chair Pose

From a standing position, bring your legs together with your feet touching. Sink your hips back like you are about to sit on a chair and bring your arms above you, holding them straight up next to your ears. Hold for 45 seconds to 1 minute. If you want to challenge yourself more, try to shift a little more weight onto your heels. This engages your core muscles and works on your balance.

mat matters

This pose requires a lot of core strength, so if you're having difficulty, you can make it easier by not sinking your hips as far down. To do this, pretend like you are trying to sit on a bar stool instead of a chair.

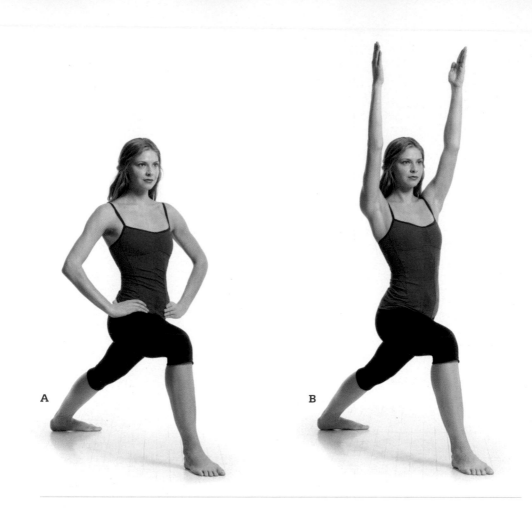

A

B

Warrior 1

Starting from the Chair Pose, come back up to a standing position. You can shake out your legs if you feel the need. **(A)** Step your left leg back about 3 feet and bend your right knee to a 90-degree angle. Try to point your back toes slightly forward while keeping your heel pressed down. **(B)** Then bring your arms up toward the ceiling. The goal in this pose is to have your thigh parallel to the floor. I want you to feel like you are trying to reach the ceiling with your fingertips as you sink down with your lower body. Keep your upper body straight and hold for 1 minute. Come back up to a standing position. Now step your right leg back 3 feet and bend your left leg to a 90-degree angle. Bring your arms straight up toward the ceiling. Hold for 1 minute. Take a second and try to notice if there was a difference between one side and the other. One of our goals, besides gaining a flat belly, is to balance out your body to prevent injury and create symmetry.

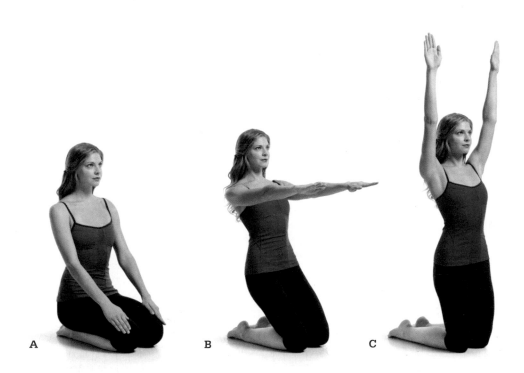

Hero Pose with a Lift

(A) Come down to the floor with your knees together and sit on your feet. Rest your hands on top of your thighs. Take a deep breath in. **(B)** On your exhale, begin to lift your arms as you raise yourself up onto your knees. **(C)** Once you are on your knees and your hands are pointed up toward the ceiling, slowly lower yourself back down to your starting position. Do this 5 times.

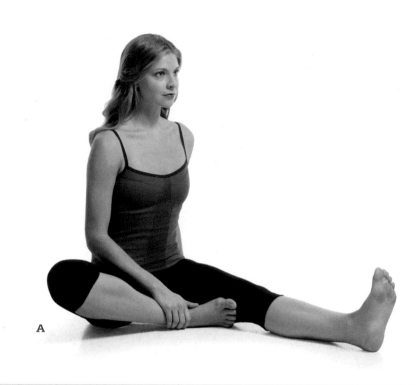

A

Seated Tree—Up and Over

Swing your legs out in front of you and shake them out. From here we are going to do one of my favorite Yoga for Your Core poses. This pose not only flattens your belly but also gets rid of your muffin top. **A** Bring your right foot to the inside of your left leg. Place your right hand on the mat or floor beside your right hip for support. **B** With your left arm, reach up and over your head toward the right side of your body and then back down to shoulder height. Make sure you're sitting up straight. Repeat this 5 times, inhaling as you reach up and exhaling as you bring your arm back down. We will be doing this pose with weights during the 4-Week Workout, so I want to make sure you get your form down now. After you have done this 5 times, switch sides. Your left foot should come to the inside of your right leg. Bring your left hand

B

beside your left hip for support, while your right hand comes up and over toward your left, and then back down to shoulder height. Do this 5 times slowly. Sitting up straight will help you focus on your core. If you can't sit up straight, you can modify the pose by not reaching up and over so far. Or you can sit up on a folded blanket, which helps to keep you from slouching.

mat matters

Try to get your foot to the inside of your thigh. If you have trouble, just bring your foot to your knee (or to your calf) to modify the pose.

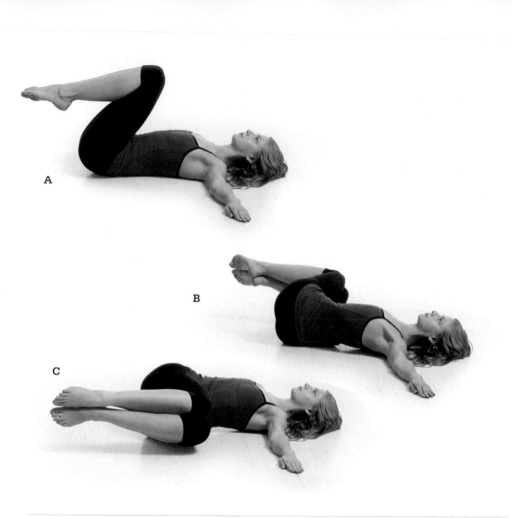

A

B

C

Windshield Wiper

A Next, bring your knees together and roll down onto your back. Bring your arms straight out so that they are parallel to your shoulders. While keeping your head and neck straight, look up at the ceiling. **B** Take a deep breath in and on your exhale, lower your legs while pointing them toward the right side of the room. Hover your legs about 2 or 3 inches from the floor. **C** Take a deep breath in and on your exhale, switch so that your legs are pointed toward the left side of the room. Do this 5 times on each side. Be sure to keep your upper back pressed to the floor. This pose works your obliques—the sides of your body. Once you've completed this pose, hug your knees into your chest and rock side to side.

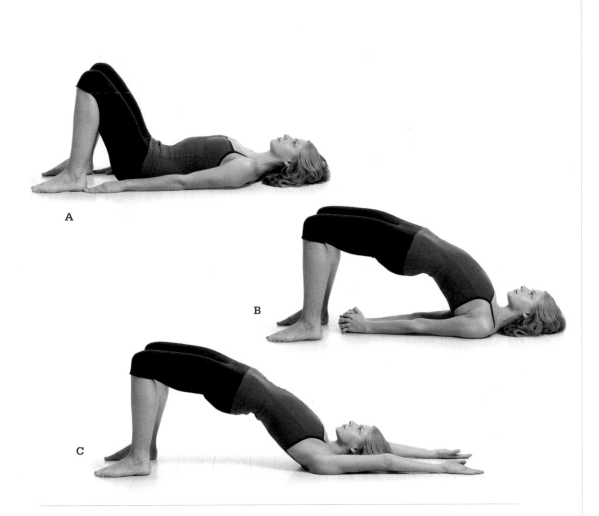

A

B

C

Bridge with a Lift

(A) While lying on your back, place your feet on the floor with your knees bent, and bring your feet hip-distance apart. Take a deep breath in. (B) On your exhale, push into your feet to lift your hips toward the ceiling. Once your hips are up, bring your arms underneath your body and clasp your hands together. Try to roll your shoulder blades together and raise your chest toward your chin while keeping your hips raised toward the ceiling. Release your arms and slowly lower your hips down to the floor. (C) Repeat, but this time bring your arms over your head. Once the back of your hands touch the floor behind your head, bring them back down to where they started. Really focus on your core/abs when you are doing this pose. Do this one more time. Once you're finished, hug your knees into your chest and rock side to side.

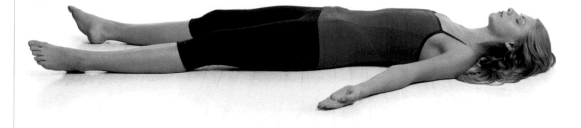

Corpse

Take a deep breath in. On your exhale, lie on the floor with your palms facing up and your eyes closed. Take a deep breath in through your nose and exhale from your mouth. Take two more deep breaths and just let your whole body relax onto the floor. Hold this pose for 2 minutes. Then roll onto your right side and push yourself up to a seated position. Take a second to evaluate how you feel. Then take a minute or two and write about your feelings in your Flat Belly Yoga! Journal (see Chapter 9 on page 177).

MOVE TO THE MUSIC

Since music is such a great motivator for working out, here are a couple of playlist suggestions to help you stay motivated during your walks and your yoga routine.

Yoga for Your Core

Song: "For the Love of Money"
Artist: The O'Jays
Album: *Ship Ahoy*
Time: 3:45

Song: "Whatcha See Is Whatcha Get"
Artist: The Dramatics
Album: *Whatcha See Is Whatcha Get*
Time: 3:57

Song: "Smiling Faces Sometimes"
Artist: The Undisputed Truth
Album: *Billboard Hot Soul Hits 1971*
Time: 3:18

Song: "Living for the City"
Artist: Stevie Wonder
Album: *Innervisions*
Time: 3:41

Heart Walk

Song: "Instant Karma"
Artist: U2
Album: *Instant Karma: The Amnesty International Campaign to Save Darfur*
Time: 3:13

Song: "Pop Song 89"
Artist: Motion City Soundtrack
Album: *Punk Goes 80's*
Time: 3:06

Song: "Hello I Love You"
Artist: The Cure
Album: *Join the Dots: B-Sides and Rarities, 1978–2001 (The Fiction Years)*
Time: 3:31

Song: "We're an American Band"
Artist: Poison
Album: *The Best of Poison: 20 Years of Rock*
Time: 3:10

Song: "Born to Be Wild"
Artist: The Cult
Album: *Electric*
Time: 3:55

A FLAT BELLY YOGA
SUCCESS STORY

Helena Ruffin

Age: 55

Pounds lost:

9

in 32 days

All-over inches lost:

11

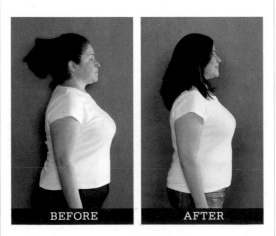

BEFORE AFTER

"I wasn't very strong," admits Helena Ruffin. After an injury left her with a broken foot and ankle, she was forced to rest and give up her workout regimen. "I was laid up for 3 months. I had gained weight, lost strength, and eventually lost interest in working out due to the pain I felt when I could walk again."

Helena knew that in order to recover properly from her injury, she had to build up her strength again and shed those extra pounds she'd gained during her time away from the gym. And she knew exactly where she needed to begin her journey: yoga. "I had never done yoga daily—at most, just a couple of times a week. I enjoyed yoga, so taking the plunge to do it daily wasn't that big of a stretch."

Because Helena was recovering from an injury, she knew she had to go at her own pace when beginning the 4-Day Jump Start. "I gave myself permission to start off slow with the goal of getting stronger every day," she says. "That was the cool part—I thought it would be difficult at first, but I felt the yoga poses become easier each day. It was a piece of cake. Well, not literally." So by the time she was ready to begin the 4-Week Workout, Helena knew she was up for the additional challenge of adding weights to her routine.

Her favorite part of the program was the structure that Flat Belly Yoga! provides. She knew she needed a plan that had a specific beginning and end in order to stay focused—and the Flat Belly Yoga! Workout fit the bill. After she completed the Jump Start, Helena had lost 2 pounds in 4 days and felt stronger and more confident than before. "I knew the plan was working for me right after the Jump Start because I could see the immediate physical results between the weight loss and feeling stronger."

Thanks to her incredible results from the Jump Start, Helena found herself excited and even more motivated for the next 4 weeks of the plan. "Every day, I found myself looking forward to the workout and thinking about the yoga program I would engage in. Even in Week 3, when I felt a bit of physical fatigue, I dragged myself to my mat and was energized by the end of the routine."

And now that she's regained her strength and dropped a full clothing size, Helena only looks to the future—a future that includes the Flat Belly Yoga! Workout. "Knowing the program, especially the Jump Start, worked so well, I can see myself using it as my go-to plan if I see a pound or two creep back, or if I need to trim down a bit more for an event," she says. "I can do yoga, follow the diet, and know the weight will come off—all from doing something I love."

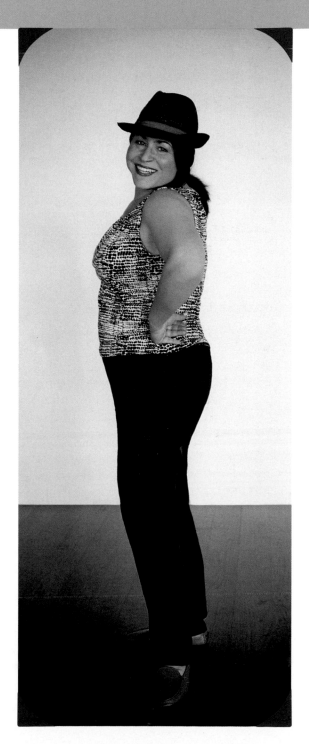

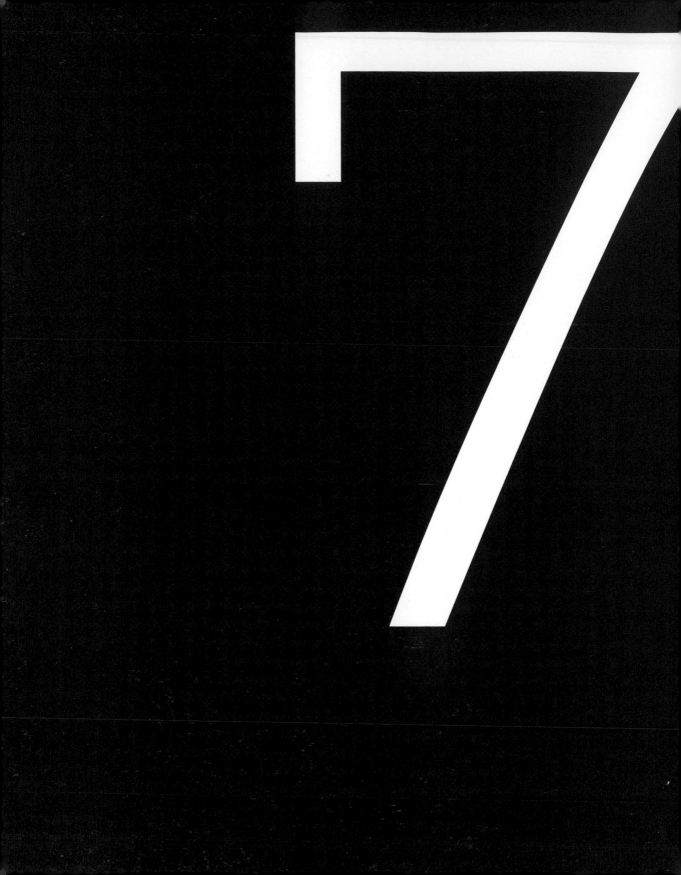

THE 4-WEEK WORKOUT

Congratulations! You've made it through the 4-Day Jump Start and now you're ready to begin the 4-Week Workout! I hope you're enjoying the positive feelings that come from working out—both the physical high, also known as an endorphin rush, and the emotional satisfaction of setting a goal and achieving it. Look at all you've accomplished in the past 4 days by making time for yourself. So before we go any further, take a minute and congratulate yourself with one more stretch: Reach your arm over your shoulder and pat yourself on the back! While it's not officially a yoga pose, it is one of the most important things you can do.

Keeping a positive attitude is the key to making it through this monthlong challenge. And maintaining this positive attitude means appreciating yourself for the challenges you've already faced. This isn't the time to be shy: By placing a high value on the time you make for yourself now, you'll continue to make yourself (and your health!) a priority throughout the next 28 days. So in 2 weeks when your friend says, "Wow, you've been working out a lot. Why can't you skip a day to come hang out with me?" you'll know the answer right away. You won't be tempted to set aside your workout because you'll feel too good about what you're accomplishing to let yourself down by missing a workout. (And by that time, you're going to look and feel so good that your friend will probably want to join you for your workouts.)

Now that you've given yourself the proper number of pats on the back (you can give yourself high fives too, although they don't have the same stretching benefit), it's time to find out what's in store for the next 4 weeks.

The Flat Belly Yoga! 4-Week Workout

The Flat Belly Yoga! 4-Week Workout incorporates weights into your yoga routine (Core+ Yoga). Combining this with your Heart Walk for cardio, this newly charged workout is designed to slim, tone, and flatten your belly—no crunches required! And even though the Core+ workouts only call for hand weights, you'll find that your lower body is getting a great workout at the same time as your upper body. So don't be surprised if you feel a little burn in your legs afterwards and see results in your lower body as well.

The workout starts with moderate-level Core+ routines and Heart Walk cardio sessions and gradually builds in intensity. The following sessions are divided into Core+ 10-, 15-, 20-, and 30-minute workouts. The intensity of each Core+ workout corresponds with your progress through the 4-Week Workout. Each week you will become stronger and have the ability to add extra poses and even hold your poses longer. So over the next 4 weeks as you progress into a more intense workout, you're going to build muscles, rev up your metabolism, and do more than take off a few pounds—you're going to turn your body into a belly-fat-reducing machine!

Start your journey by charting your course through the 4-Week Workout on page 187. Take a look at your calendar and decide when and where you're going to perform each workout. Each routine is accompanied by step-by-step instructions that include the total time and the relative intensity, which will help you plan out your weeks. Hopefully you have learned more about your workout preferences from completing the 4-Day Jump Start and already have a spot and time of day in mind. Whatever your preferences, try to schedule your walks (preferably beforehand) along with your Core+ workouts.

For now, just pencil in your choices and schedule for the first week. You might want to make changes or adjustments once you get going. Keep in mind that you're using a pencil so you can adjust your schedule, not so you can erase it! Don't be flexible to the point of skipping your workouts. Remember: You have to make time for yourself. If you find that this is becoming difficult, try charting your progress. This not only helps you stay on track with your workout, but also forces you to acknowledge and feel good about the effort you're making to take care of yourself. And you'll only get better at charting your progress and planning your workouts as you move through each week of the plan.

It's really important to me for you to have fun during these 4 weeks because if you're not having fun, you won't continue to work out. But if you take the time to find the places in your week where your workout sessions fit just right, you'll make working out a part of your life—for 28 days and long after. Get ready to launch into your Flat Belly Yoga! 4-Week Workout!

PLAY IT SAFE Remember to take your workout at your own pace. If you're feeling that the workout is too much for you, lower the intensity. Still do your workout—just not as hard.

(continued on page 108)

The 4-Week Flat Belly Yoga!

Week	Day 1	Day 2	Day 3	Day 4	Day 5
1	**Fat Blast Walk** 30 minutes • 3-minute warm-up • 25-minute fast pace • 2-minute cooldown	**Calorie Torch Walk** 25 minutes • 3-minute warm-up • 4-minute fast pace with 1-minute pick-me-ups (repeat 4x) • 2-minute cooldown	**Fat Blast Walk** 30 minutes • 3-minute warm-up • 25-minute fast pace • 2-minute cooldown	**Calorie Torch Walk** 25 minutes • 3-minute warm-up • 4-minute fast pace with 1-minute pick-me-ups (repeat 4x) • 2-minute cooldown	**Fat Blast Walk** 30 minutes • 3-minute warm-up • 25-minute fast pace • 2-minute cooldown
	Core+ 10-Minute Workout	Core+ 10-Minute Workout	Core+ 10-Minute Workout	Core+ 10-Minute Workout	Core+ 10-Minute Workout
2	**Fat Blast Walk** 45 minutes • 3-minute warm-up • 40-minute fast pace • 2-minute cooldown	**Calorie Torch Walk** 35 minutes • 3-minute warm-up • 4-minute fast pace with 1-minute pick-me-ups (repeat 6x) • 2-minute cooldown	**Fat Blast Walk** 45 minutes • 3-minute warm-up • 40-minute fast pace • 2-minute cooldown	**Calorie Torch Walk** 35 minutes • 3-minute warm-up • 4-minute fast pace with 1-minute pick-me-ups (repeat 6x) • 2-minute cooldown	**Fat Blast Walk** 45 minutes • 3-minute warm-up • 40-minute fast pace • 2-minute cooldown
	Core+ 15-Minute Workout	Core+ 15-Minute Workout	Core+ 15-Minute Workout	Core+ 15-Minute Workout	Core+ 15-Minute Workout
3	**Fat Blast Walk** 60 minutes • 3-minute warm-up • 55-minute fast pace • 2-minute cooldown	**Calorie Torch Walk** 45 minutes • 3-minute warm-up • 4-minute fast pace with 1-minute pick-me-ups (repeat 8x) • 2-minute cooldown	**Fat Blast Walk** 60 minutes • 3-minute warm-up • 55-minute fast pace • 2-minute cooldown	**Calorie Torch Walk** 45 minutes • 3-minute warm-up • 4-minute fast pace with 1-minute pick-me-ups (repeat 8x) • 2-minute cooldown	**Fat Blast Walk** 60 minutes • 3-minute warm-up • 55-minute fast pace • 2-minute cooldown
	Core+ 20-Minute Workout	Core+ 20-Minute Workout	Core+ 20-Minute Workout	Core+ 20-Minute Workout	Core+ 20-Minute Workout
4	**Fat Blast Walk** 60 minutes • 3-minute warm-up • 55-minute fast pace • 2-minute cooldown	**Calorie Torch Walk** 45 minutes • 3-minute warm-up • 4-minute fast pace with 1-minute pick-me-ups (repeat 8x) • 2-minute cooldown	**Fat Blast Walk** 60 minutes • 3-minute warm-up • 55-minute fast pace • 2-minute cooldown	**Calorie Torch Walk** 45 minutes • 3-minute warm-up • 4-minute fast pace with 1-minute pick-me-ups (repeat 8x) • 2-minute cooldown	**Fat Blast Walk** 60 minutes • 3-minute warm-up • 55-minute fast pace • 2-minute cooldown
	Core+ 30-Minute Workout	Core+ 30-Minute Workout	Core+ 30-Minute Workout	Core+ 30-Minute Workout	Core+ 30-Minute Workout

Workout Plan

Day 6	Day 7
Calorie Torch Walk 25 minutes • 3-minute warm-up • 4-minute fast pace with 1-minute pick-me-ups (repeat 4x) • 2-minute cooldown	Rest
Core+ 10-Minute Workout	
Calorie Torch Walk 35 minutes • 3-minute warm-up • 4-minute fast pace with 1-minute pick-me-ups (repeat 6x) • 2-minute cooldown	Rest
Core+ 15-Minute Workout	
Calorie Torch Walk 45 minutes • 3-minute warm-up • 4-minute fast pace with 1-minute pick-me-ups (repeat 8x) • 2-minute cooldown	Rest
Core+ 20-Minute Workout	
Calorie Torch Walk 45 minutes • 3-minute warm-up • 4-minute fast pace with 1-minute pick-me-ups (repeat 8x) • 2-minute cooldown	Rest
Core+ 30-Minute Workout	

mat motivation

My Toughest 4-Week Challenge

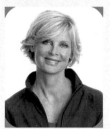

Four weeks really isn't a lot of time, but when it comes to making a commitment and sticking with it, a single month may seem like forever. That can be true even for a pretty disciplined person like me, which I discovered the hard way a few years ago.

The project was my first book, *The No Om Zone*. I had done a lot of things in my life, but writing a book wasn't one of them. Giving me a new yoga workout to master was no problem. But asking me to come up with 75,000 words? That seemed like a big stretch. And that was before I knew it would take several weeks of 16-hour days at the keyboard to make my deadline.

Given my career choice, it's safe to say that I'm not the type of person who likes to sit in front of a computer all day. Yet here I was, writing a book about yoga, but unable to go for a walk, let alone get to the studio for a real workout. How's that for irony?

Aside from the crazy hours, I wasn't convinced I had a book in me. Yes, I had strong opinions and a lot of knowledge about yoga. But did that necessarily make me an author? I wasn't so sure.

So here's what I did: I came up with a plan, which is always my first step when I need to overcome a challenge. I knew what my goal was, and I also knew that I had a firm deadline, which is always a good source of motivation and discipline. So then I created a set amount of time to write each day, both to give me a clear path and to keep me from bolting from my desk.

And guess what? I wrote the book and made the deadline. True, I had to skip my workouts for a while—something I almost never do. But the book was my priority and other things simply had to give.

That's exactly how you have to approach the 4-Week Workout, or any exercise routine, for that matter. If you decide to make it a priority, something else may have to go by the wayside. That's just reality. But the trade-off is worth it, in so many ways, as you'll find out in the next 4 weeks.

Core+ 10-Minute Workout Routine

Now that you're familiar with the yoga poses from the Jump Start, we are going to make it a little more challenging by adding 3-pound weights. If you need a refresher, everything you need to know about combining weights with yoga is laid out for you in Chapter 2 on page 17.

When you're ready to begin, place your weights at the top of your mat, or if you're not using a mat, on the floor in front of you so you can easily reach them. Yoga is a great strength-training exercise, and by incorporating weights, we are really going to focus on sculpting and toning your body. If you become too tired, you can always just put your weights down and do the workout without them. But try to use them as much as you can: The Core+ workouts are designed to build lean muscle mass quickly, so you'll see faster results by incorporating the weights as often as possible.

1 Warm-Up/Breath Work
p. 88

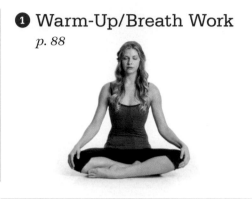

4 Chair Pose
p. 112

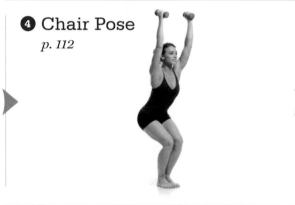

7 Seated Tree with a Lift
p. 115

10 Corpse
p. 98

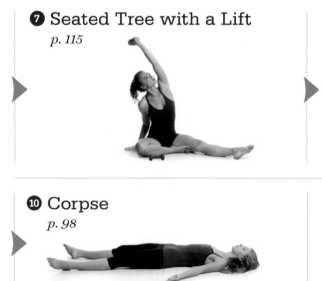

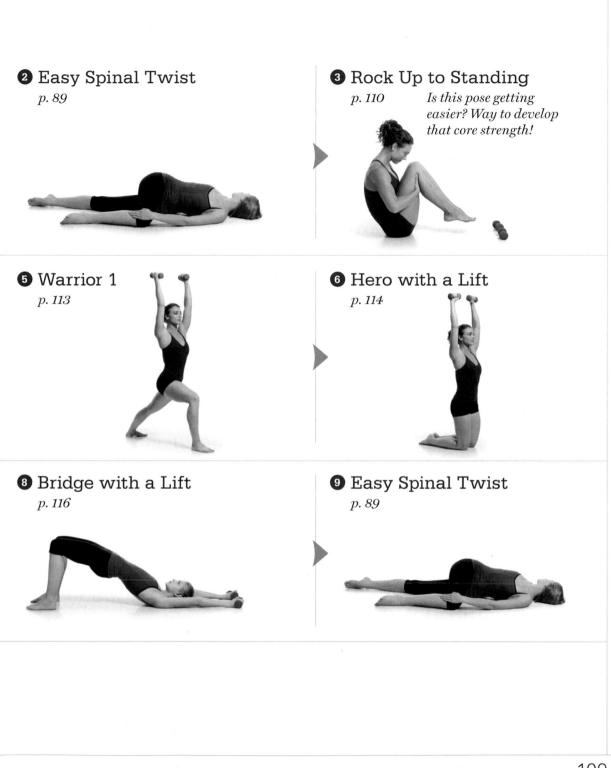

2 Easy Spinal Twist
p. 89

3 Rock Up to Standing
p. 110   *Is this pose getting easier? Way to develop that core strength!*

5 Warrior 1
p. 113

6 Hero with a Lift
p. 114

8 Bridge with a Lift
p. 116

9 Easy Spinal Twist
p. 89

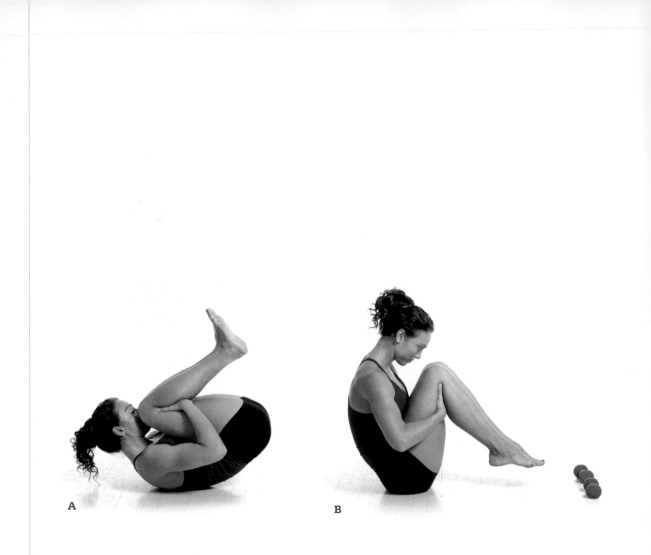

A

B

Rock Up to Standing

A Begin by lying on your back with your knees pulled into your chest. **B** Rock up and back from your shoulders to your hips, getting up the momentum to rock up to a standing position. (Remember that this position is hard even for someone who has been practicing yoga for a while, so don't get discouraged.) You can make this easier by using your hands to help push you up off the floor. Take in a deep breath and on your exhale, bend forward at your hips. **C** Bend your knees and grab hold of your weights. Take in a deep breath. As you exhale, slowly roll up to standing one vertebra at a time, bringing up your head last. **D** Extend your arms up toward the ceiling while holding onto your weights.

C

D

mat matters

Since you are holding onto your weights, this might be challenging. Try engaging your core muscles to help you stay in this pose. And make sure not to let your arms fall.

Chair Pose

From a standing position, bring your legs together with your feet touching. Sink your hips back like you are about to sit down. With your weights in your hands, keep your arms up beside your ears. Hold for 45 seconds to 1 minute.

mat matters

Want to challenge yourself a little more? Try to sink deeper into the pose while holding onto the weights.

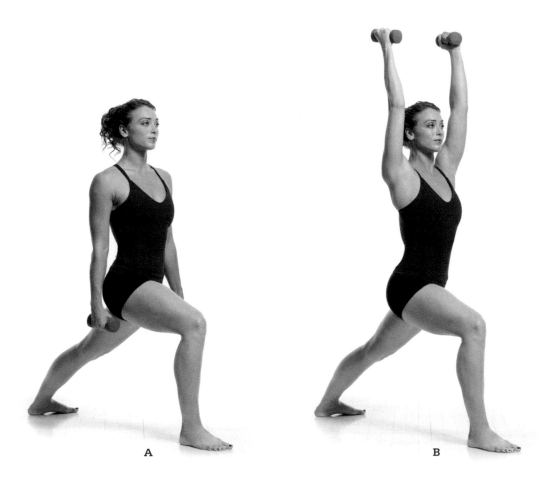

A

B

Warrior 1

Begin from a standing position. You can shake out your arms and legs if needed.
A Holding onto your weights, step your left leg back about 3 feet and bend
your right knee to a 90-degree angle. **B** Bring your arms up toward the ceiling.
(I want you to feel like you are trying to reach the ceiling with your weights as you
sink down with your lower body.) Try to keep your upper body straight. Make sure
your hips and shoulders are squared (aligned and facing forward). Hold for 1 minute.
Come back up to a standing position. Shake it out and switch sides. Step your right
leg back about 3 feet and bend your left leg to a 90-degree angle. Square your
hips and shoulders. Bring your weights straight up to the ceiling. Hold for 1 minute.
Stand up and shake out your legs.

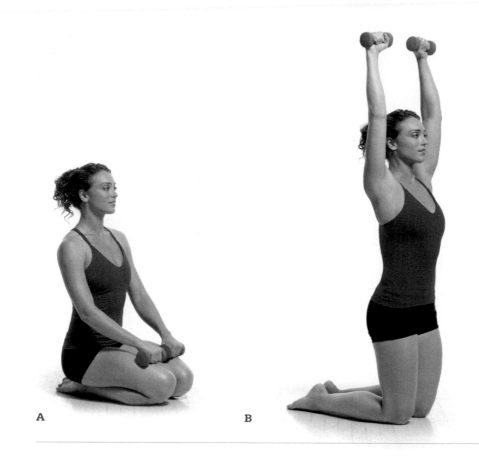

A   B

Hero with a Lift

A Come down to the floor with your knees together and sit on your feet. While holding your weights, bring your hands to the top of your thighs, palms facing down.

B Take a deep breath in and on your exhale, come up onto your knees, bringing your weights over your head, straight up to the ceiling. Then slowly lower them back down, using your core strength, and sit back on your feet. Keep your palms facing forward as you lift. Do this 5 times. This pose stretches the front of the body and strengthens the lower back, really toning your belly!

mat matters

Don't swing your weights to get momentum. Instead, use your quadriceps to pull your body forward and up.

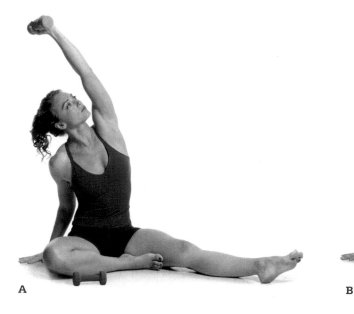

A

B

Seated Tree with a Lift

This is a great pose to help get rid of "love handles." Seated on the floor, swing your legs out in front of you and shake them out. Bring your right foot to the inside of your left thigh. If this is too difficult, try placing your foot closer to your knee. Place your right hand on the floor beside your right hip. **A** Grab a weight with your left hand and then reach up with your left arm. Stretch your left arm toward the right side of your body without turning your shoulders or leaning forward. **B** Then bend your left elbow and bring it down to shoulder height. Repeat this 5 times, inhaling as you reach up and exhaling as you bring your arm down. Now switch sides and repeat the entire sequence 5 times on the other side. When finished, place your weights on the floor by your hips, bring your knees together, and roll down onto your back.

mat matters

Make sure you're sitting up straight during this pose. This will engage your core and reduce the tendency to slouch.

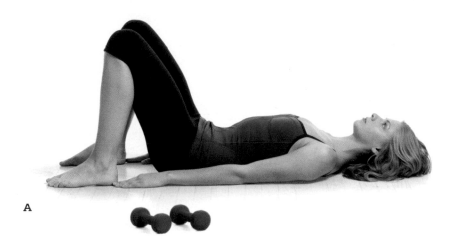

A

Bridge with a Lift

A Begin lying on your mat with your knees bent and your feet hip-distance apart. Reach down with your fingertips and try to reach your heels. If you can't reach your heels, walk your feet a little closer to your body. **B** Take in a deep breath and as you exhale, push your feet down onto the floor to lift your hips up toward the ceiling. Once your hips are up, bring your arms underneath you and clasp your hands together. Try to roll your shoulder blades together, which will stretch your chest muscles. Raise your chest up toward your chin. Release your arms and slowly lower yourself down onto the floor. We are going to do this 2 more times using your weights. **C** Grab your weights and extend your arms over your head as you lift your hips to the ceiling. Once the back of your hands touch the floor behind your head, bring them back down to where you started as you lower your hips back to the floor. This stretches the front of your body, your core, while strengthening your lower back, so really focus on your abs during this pose. Once you're finished, release your weights. Hug your knees into your chest and rock side to side.

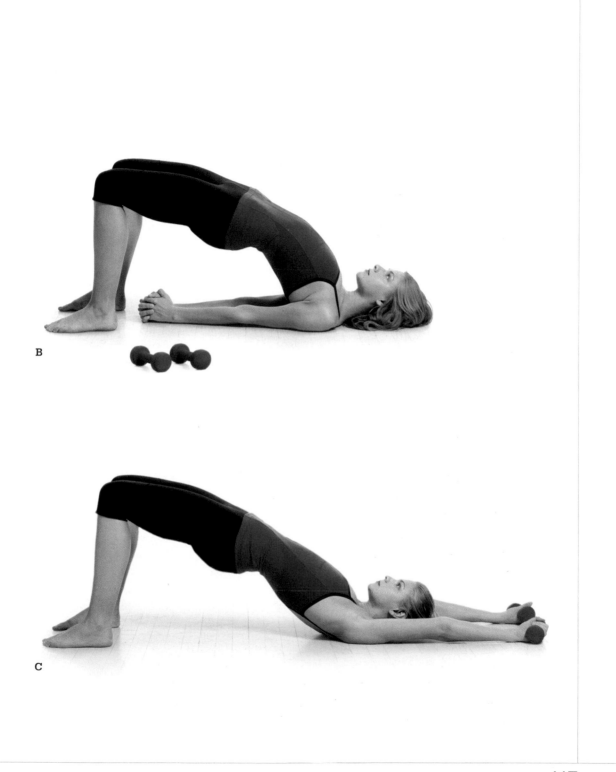

B

C

Core+ 15-Minute Workout Routine

As you're going through this workout, it's important to take note of how long you are holding the poses on each side so that you're getting a balanced workout. (Sometimes we hold poses longer on our easier side.)

Afterwards, take a second and notice how you feel. I hope you feel better than when you started. (Remember: Take a minute or two and write down how you feel in your Flat Belly Yoga! Journal, found in Chapter 9 on page 177.)

❶ Warm-Up/Breath Work

p. 88

Use your core to sit up straight. This should be getting easier.

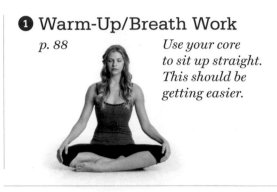

❹ Chair Pose

p. 112

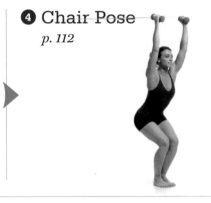

❼ Upright Rows

p. 120

❽ Seated Tree with a Lift

p. 115

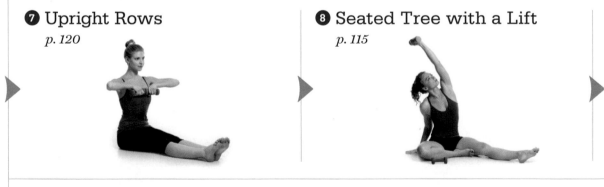

⓫ Easy Spinal Twist

p. 89

Hold for 45 seconds. (You'll need this pose—especially after doing Boat with a Burn!)

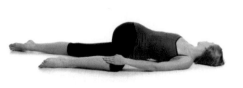

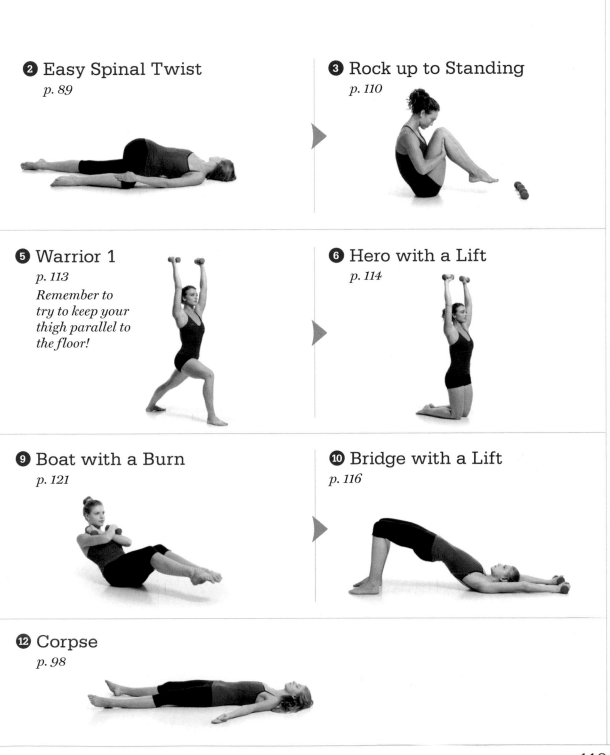

❷ Easy Spinal Twist
p. 89

❸ Rock up to Standing
p. 110

❺ Warrior 1
p. 113
Remember to try to keep your thigh parallel to the floor!

❻ Hero with a Lift
p. 114

❾ Boat with a Burn
p. 121

❿ Bridge with a Lift
p. 116

⓬ Corpse
p. 98

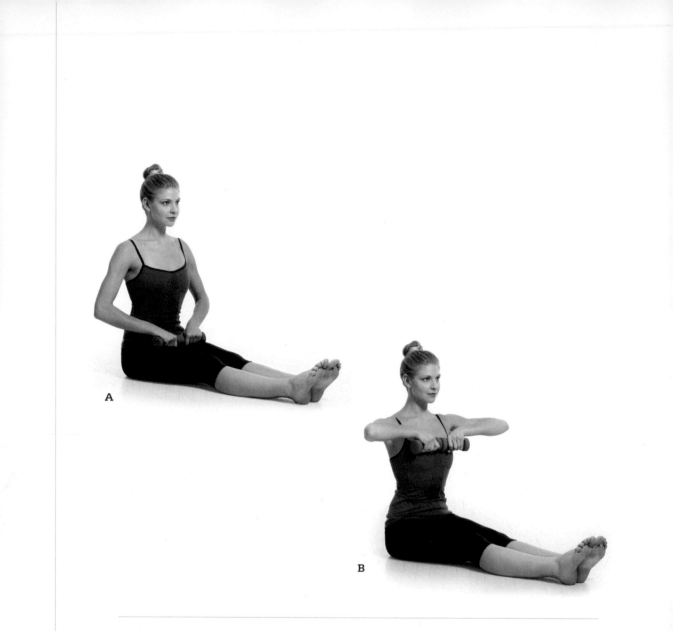

A

B

Upright Rows

Sitting on the floor, swing your legs out in front of you and shake them out. (A) From here, bring your weights to the top of your thighs for some Upright Rows. You can keep your legs together or, if it's hard to sit up straight, place your legs wide apart. (B) Lift your weights up to your chest, making sure to keep the ends of your weights together. Your elbows should be out to your sides. Hold it for about 10 seconds, then release them back to your thighs. Let's do this 5 times.

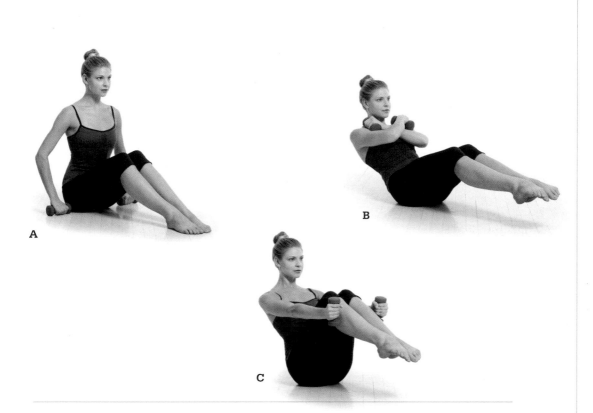

A

B

C

Boat with a Burn

This pose on its own is hard, and with weights it's a killer! **A** Begin in a seated position with your knees bent and your feet on the floor. **B** Bring your knees together and raise your feet up off the floor. Grab your weights and cross your arms at your chest. Slowly lower your back a few inches, keeping your knees slightly bent, then come back up. **C** Once you are back up, straighten your arms and bring your weights out alongside your knees. Hold for 10 seconds. Next, bring the weights across your chest and lower back down again. (Note: If you're having difficulty completing this pose with the weights, you can place them on the floor or simply don't lower yourself as far. Customize it to fit your level.) Do this 5 times. Then bring your knees into your chest and roll down onto the mat. Hug your knees into your chest and rock side to side to release your lower back.

mat matters

When you are lowering down and coming back up, you can straighten your legs if you want an extra challenge.

Core+ 20-Minute Workout Routine

This workout incorporates several new poses designed to target your belly and take your workout to a whole new level. Take your time when you're doing these poses—slower movements help engage your abdominal muscles even more. As your workouts become progressively harder, you can come to the Child's Pose (see page 144) at any point during your workout to take a break if you get too tired.

❶ Breath Work Stretch
p. 129

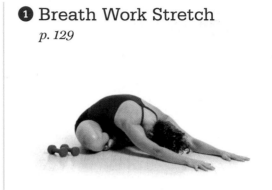

❹ Standing Forward Bend
p. 132

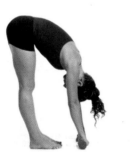

❺ Chair with Overhead Shoulder Presses/ Triceps Extensions
p. 133

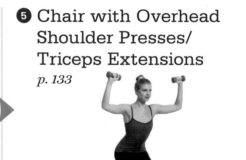

❼ Warrior 1 with Flow
p. 138

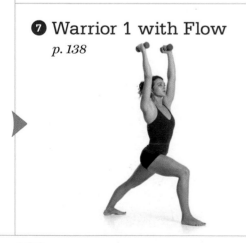

❽ Core+ Flow
p. 134

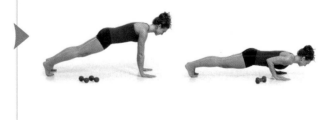

2 Easy Spinal Twist
p. 89

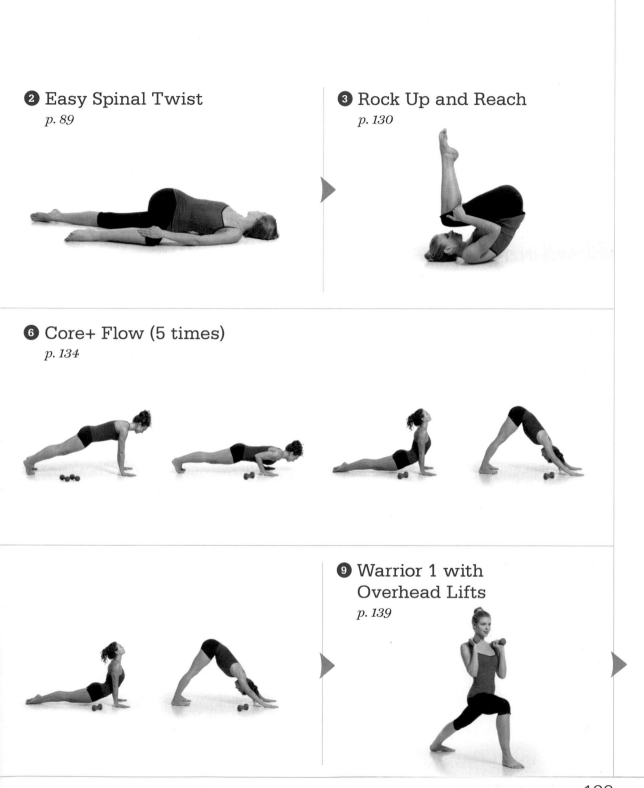

3 Rock Up and Reach
p. 130

6 Core+ Flow (5 times)
p. 134

9 Warrior 1 with Overhead Lifts
p. 139

Core+ 20-Minute Workout Routine *(cont.)*

❿ Warrior 2 with Biceps Curls
p. 140

⓫ Core+ Flow
p. 134

⓭ Warrior 2 with Biceps Curls
p. 140

⓮ Core+ Flow
p. 134

⓰ Warrior 2 with Mini-Lifts
p. 142

⓱ Side Angle with Lat Rows
p. 143

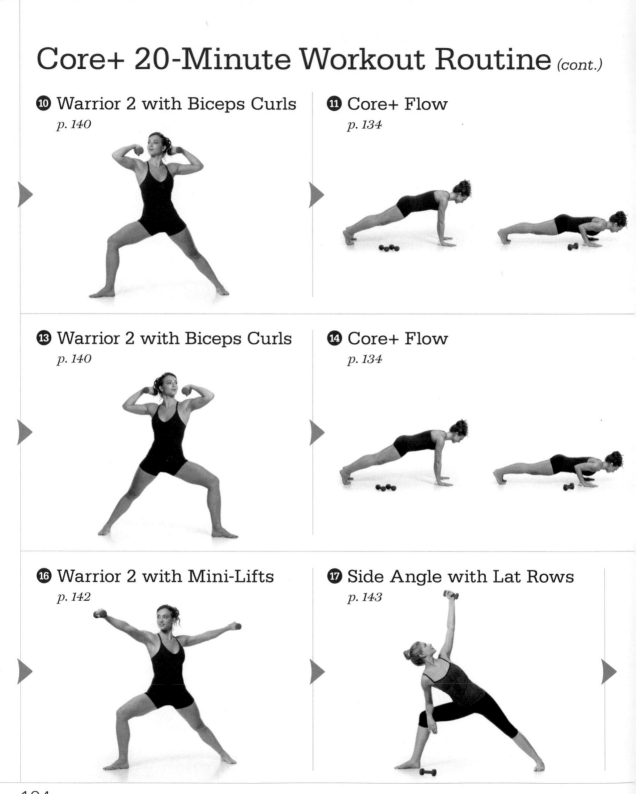

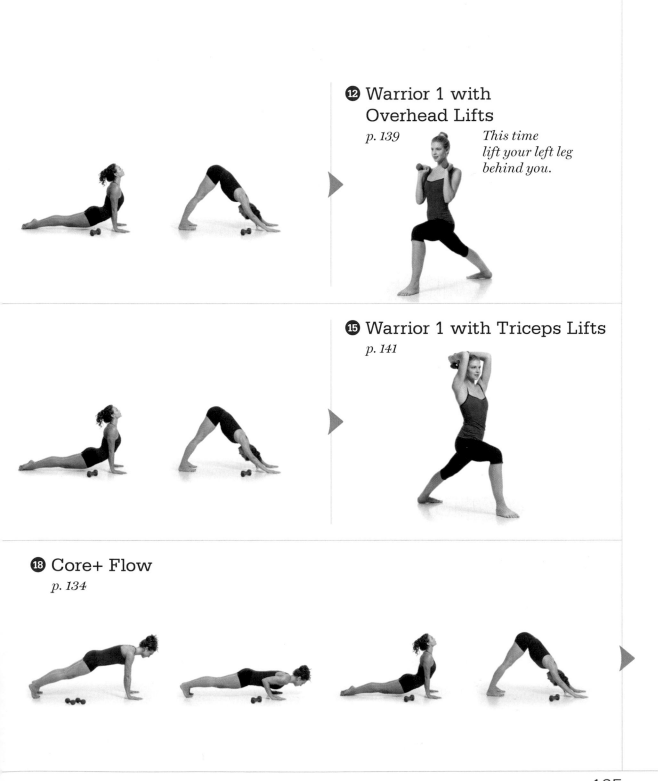

12 Warrior 1 with
Overhead Lifts

p. 139

*This time
lift your left leg
behind you.*

15 Warrior 1 with Triceps Lifts

p. 141

18 Core+ Flow

p. 134

Core+ 20-Minute Workout Routine *(cont.)*

⑲ Warrior 1 with Triceps Lifts

p. 141

*This time lift your
left leg behind you.*

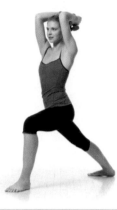

㉒ Core+ Flow

p. 134

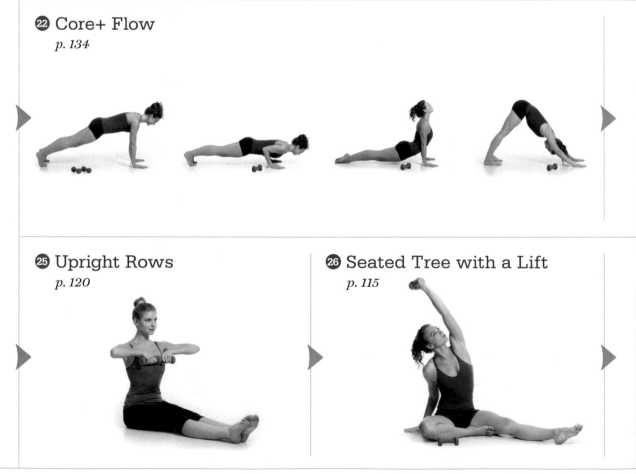

㉕ Upright Rows

p. 120

㉖ Seated Tree with a Lift

p. 115

20 Warrior 2 with Mini-Lifts
p. 142

21 Side Angle with Lat Rows
p. 143

23 Child's Pose
p. 144

24 Hero with a Lift
p. 114

27 Cobbler with Chest Fly
p. 145

28 Boat with a Burn
p. 121

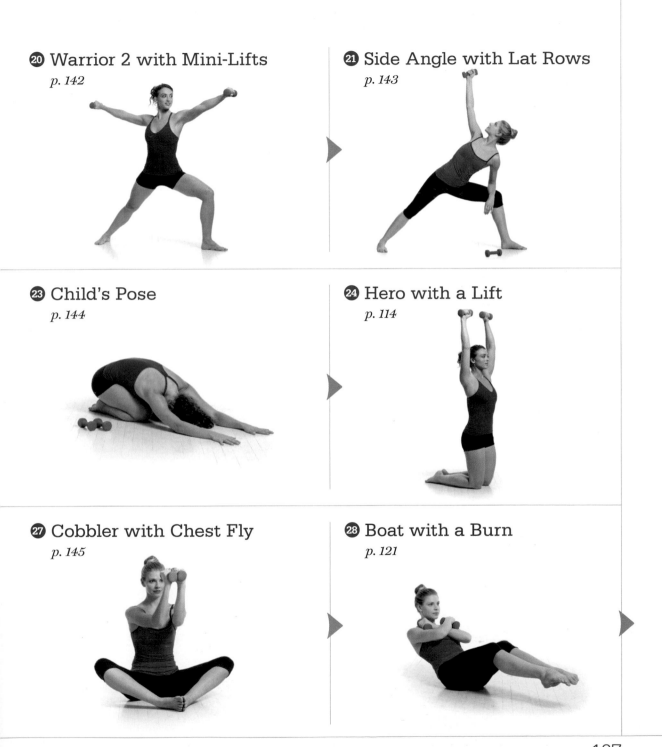

Core+ 20-Minute Workout Routine *(cont.)*

㉙ Dead Bug with Chest Press
p. 146

㉚ Advanced Bridge with a Lift
p. 147

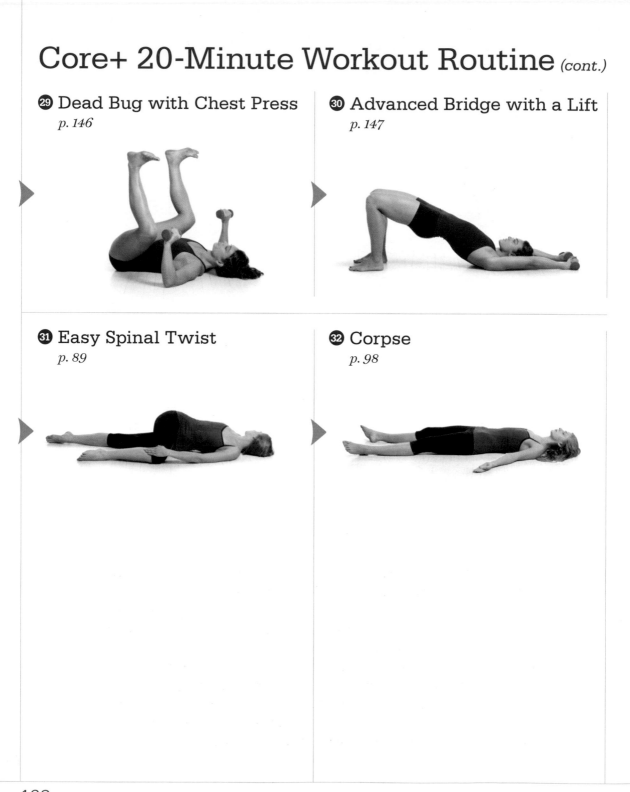

㉛ Easy Spinal Twist
p. 89

㉜ Corpse
p. 98

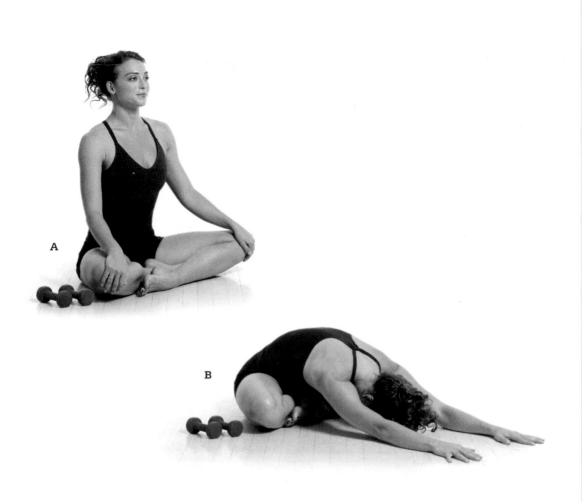

A

B

Breath Work Stretch

A Place your weights on the floor. Sit in an easy cross-legged position with one leg in front of the other. Take in a deep breath through your nose and let it out through your mouth. Let's do that 2 more times. Since we are increasing your workout, I'm going to add an extra lower back stretch to your breath work. **B** So from here, walk your hands out in front of you far enough to feel a little stretch in your lower back and hips. Lower your head so that you feel a nice stretch in your neck and shoulders. Hold for 30 seconds. Take in a deep breath and as you exhale, walk your hands back up and switch sides. Cross your legs in the opposite direction, and then walk your hands out in front of you. Hold for 30 seconds. Then take in a deep breath and walk your hands back up as you exhale. Bring your knees together and roll down onto your back.

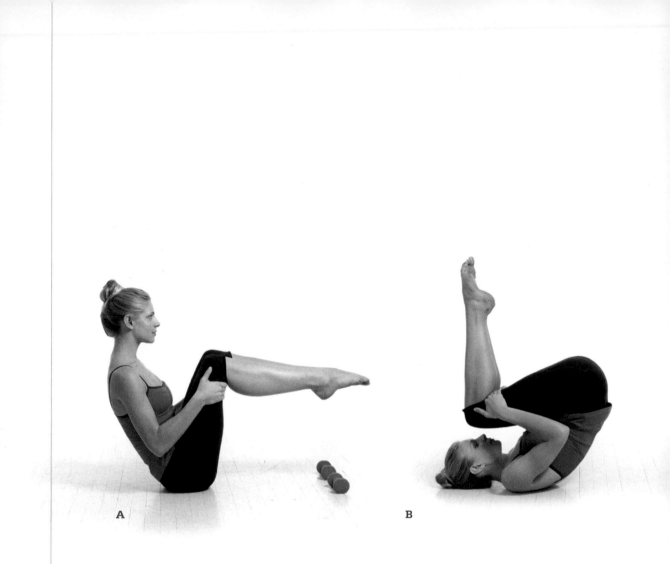

A   B

Rock Up and Reach

Ⓐ Sitting up, bring your knees together with your hands supporting the back of your knees. Ⓑ Rock back and forth from your shoulders to your hips. Do this 4 or 5 times and Rock Up to Standing (p. 110). Ⓒ Once you're standing, spread your feet about hip distance apart and bend down to pick up your weights. Ⓓ Holding your weights, stand back up and reach up toward the ceiling with both arms. Now, reach up a little farther with your right hand, and then with your left.

C

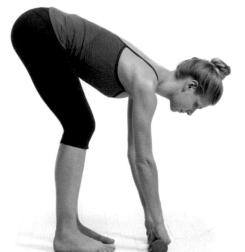

mat matters

You can take this into a little backbend by bending backwards a few inches, which will help stretch your core muscles. Be careful not to stretch too far since this is a warm-up pose.

D

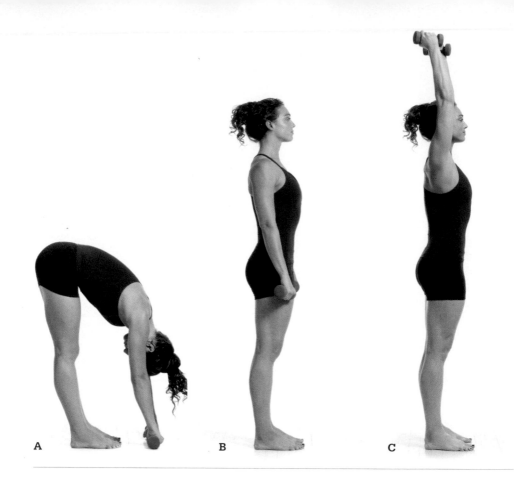

A   B   C

Standing Forward Bend

Come to a standing position. Take in a deep breath. Bend forward as you exhale and clasp opposite elbows. You can shake your head from side to side to release any tension in your neck. Hold for 20 seconds. **A** Release your arms and grab your weights. **B** Bend your knees and slowly roll up to a standing position. **C** Bring your weights straight out in front of you and reach up toward the ceiling. Once you are standing up straight, bring your legs together so that your feet are touching.

mat matters

If your lower back or hamstrings are tight, you can bend your knees a little as you hinge forward.

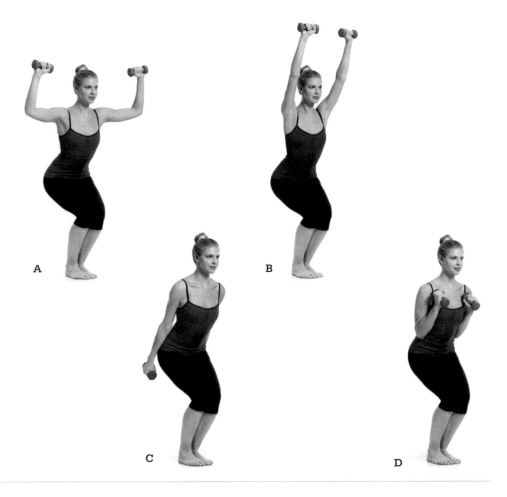

A

B

C

D

Chair with Overhead Shoulder Presses/Triceps Extensions

A Holding your weights, sink down into the Chair Pose (p. 112). To begin the Overhead Shoulder Presses, bring your elbows up to shoulder level with your palms facing forward. **B** Then lift your weights up toward the ceiling and then slowly lower them back down to shoulder level. Do this 5 times. When you are finished, hold onto your weights and rest them on your shoulders. Keep your knees bent. From here we are going to do the Triceps Extensions. **C** While still holding your weights, extend your arms behind your back. **D** Now bring your weights up to your chest, keeping your elbows in so that they're touching your rib cage. Your thighs may be burning, but hang in there. You can engage your core to help with balance. Do this 5 times slowly, then stand up. Shake out your arms and legs. Now, that's a workout!

Core+ Flow

The Core+ Flow consists of the following poses: Plank, Hover, Upward Facing Dog, and Downward Facing Dog. Doing just these poses alone will work up a sweat! And that's exactly what we are going to do. Remember that the Core+ Flow takes a lot of core strength, and the poses are not the easiest to do. But it will all be worth it when you see the results—a flat belly is on the way!

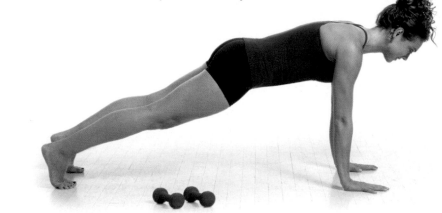

Plank Pose

Place your weights on the floor (or your mat) and lower yourself to your hands and knees. Bring your hands under your shoulders so that your shoulders, elbows, and wrists form a straight line. Extend your legs so that your body looks like the top of a push-up. Your feet should be hip-distance apart, with your toes tucked under. Make sure your body is as flat as a board by lifting the front of your thighs and pressing back through your heels. (Your hips shouldn't be higher or lower than the rest of your body.) Hold for at least 10 seconds. The strength to hold this pose comes mostly from your core, so as you're doing it, keep thinking to yourself, "I'm flattening my belly."

mat matters

If you're having trouble holding the pose during your first few attempts, you can always modify it by dropping down to your knees.

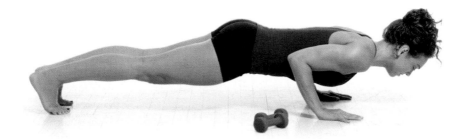

Hover Pose

Keeping your legs straight (or your knees bent) and toes tucked under, slowly lower your chest down and hover about 5 inches above the floor. Try to hold this pose for a few seconds.

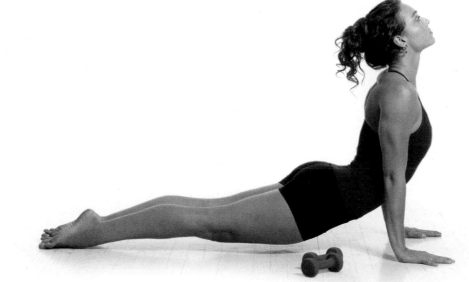

Upward Facing Dog

Next, with your legs stretched out behind you, scoop your chest forward and up by straightening your arms. Your chest should now be in line with your shoulders with most of your weight focused on your hands. Hold for 15 to 20 seconds.

Downward Facing Dog

Engaging your core muscles, pull yourself back into an inverted V shape by keeping your heels down and lifting your butt up toward the ceiling. Hold for 30 seconds.

mat matters

Let's do a quick Downward Facing Dog form check! Make sure your heels are pressed toward the floor. This will provide a good stretch for your hamstrings.

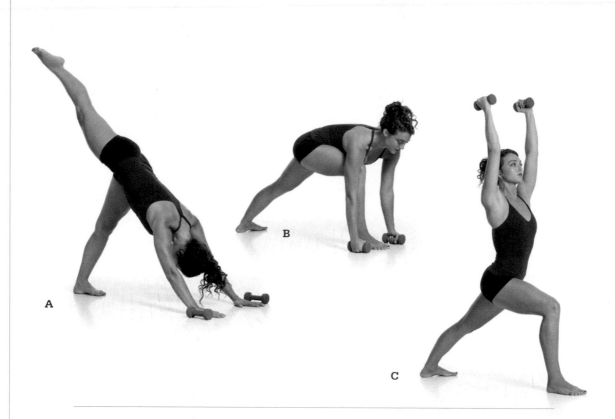

Warrior 1
with Flow

A Beginning from Downward Facing Dog, lift your right leg behind you. **B** Take in a deep breath and as you exhale, swing your right foot down and through your hands. Drop your back heel to the floor and then grab your weights. **C** Slowly lift your arms straight up toward the ceiling. Hold this pose for 30 seconds. Take in a deep breath and as you exhale, bring your weights down to the floor and place them at the top of your mat. Repeat the sequence, switching legs. When you're finished, bring your weights down and place them at the top of your mat.

mat matters

Make sure your hips and shoulders are squared to the front of the room and your front knee is in line with your ankle.

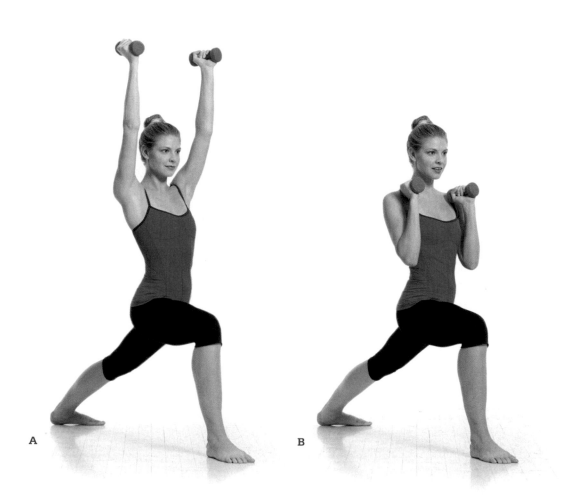

A

B

Warrior 1 with Overhead Lifts

Beginning from Downward Facing Dog, lift your right leg behind you. Swing your foot down through your hands and drop your back heel to the floor. Grab your weights and move into a Warrior 1 stance. **A** Once you're steady, lift your arms up toward the ceiling. **B** Bend your elbows and bring your weights down to shoulder height, then raise them back up. Make sure to keep your elbows in and palms facing each other. Do this 5 times, slowly, inhaling as you lift your weights and exhaling as your lower them back down. Afterwards, rest your weights on your shoulders while holding onto them.

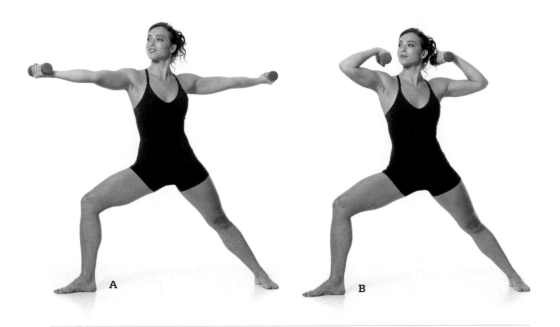

A

B

Warrior 2 with Biceps Curls

Begin in Warrior 1. Your legs should remain in place as you slowly shift your hips and shoulders toward the left side of the room so that your right arm is in line with your right knee. Make sure your right knee stays in line with your right ankle. **A** Holding onto your weights, extend your arms out with your palms facing the ceiling. **B** Then lift your hands up toward your shoulders and lower them back down again, slowly. Do this 5 times. When you're finished, rest your weights on your shoulders as you return to Warrior 1. Bring your arms up toward the ceiling and hold for 30 seconds. From here bring your weights to the floor.

mat
matters

When doing the Biceps Curls, try to keep your arms at shoulder height.

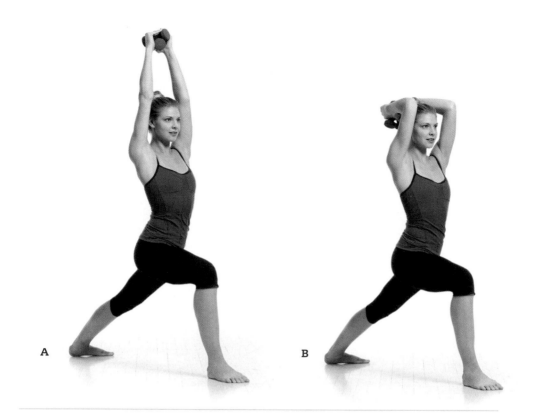

A

B

Warrior 1 with Triceps Lifts

Starting from Downward Facing Dog, lift your right leg behind you. Swing your foot down through your hands and drop your back heel to the floor. Grab your weights and move into a Warrior 1 stance. **A** Once you're steady, lift your arms up toward the ceiling for the Triceps Lifts. **B** While holding your weights over your head, bring your hands together and slowly lower them behind your head. Then lift your weights back up toward the ceiling. Do this 5 times, inhaling as you lift your weights up and exhaling as your lower them down. When you've completed the 5 reps, rest your weights on your shoulders.

mat matters

Try to keep your elbows in by your head. If your elbows are far away from your head, you'll be working your chest muscles instead of your core.

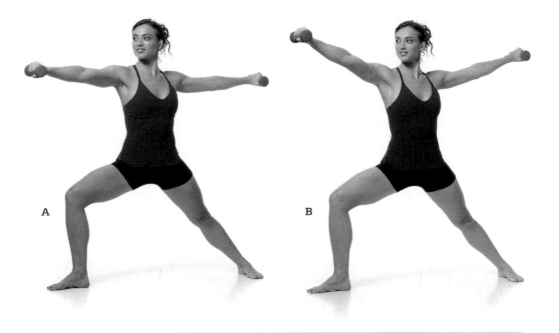

A

B

Warrior 2
with Mini-Lifts

Begin in Warrior 1. Your legs should remain
in place as you slowly shift your hips and
shoulders to the left side of the room.
Bring your right arm toward the front of
the room and your left arm toward the
back of the room at shoulder height, with
your palms facing the floor. **A** To perform the Mini-Lifts, your arms should be
fully extended at shoulder height. **B** Lift
them up a few inches and hold for a few
seconds before lowering them back down to
shoulder level. Do this 5 times. (If this is too
difficult at first, try to do the Mini-Lifts without
the weights.)

mat matters

Check to make sure you're
doing this pose correctly.
Keeping your back leg
straight offers
stability.

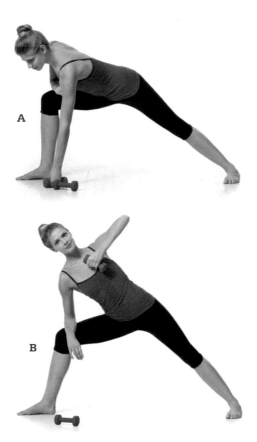

Side Angle with Lat Rows

(A) From here bring your right elbow to your right knee and your left hand to the floor. Now grab a weight. **(B)** Bring it up to your chest, making sure your elbow is pointing up toward the ceiling. **(C)** Pause for a second before lifting the weight straight up toward the ceiling. Hold for 10 seconds. Take in a deep breath and exhale as you lower your weight back down to your chest. Pause, and then lower your weight to the floor. Keep your core engaged to help stabilize your body. Do this 5 times.

mat matters

To prevent back pain, make sure your arm doesn't drop down behind your head.

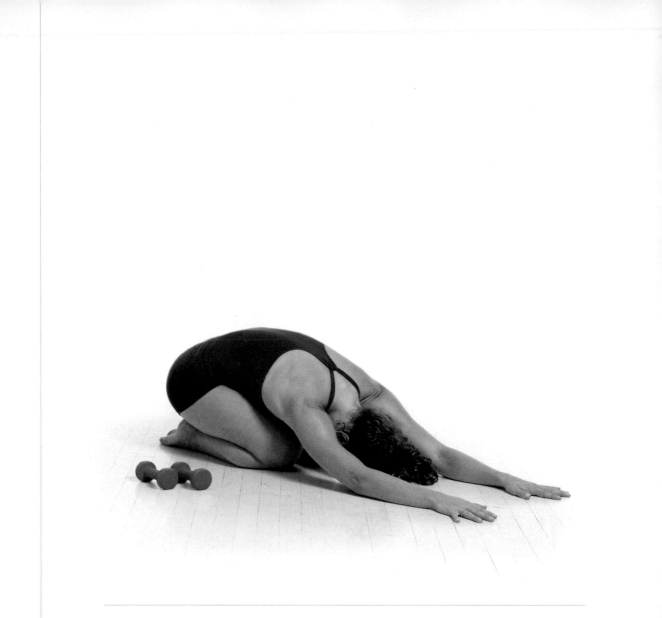

Child's Pose

Kneel onto the floor and bring your knees together. Rest your chest on your thighs, with your arms stretched out in front of you, resting on the floor. Let your forehead drop to the floor. Hold this pose for 30 seconds.

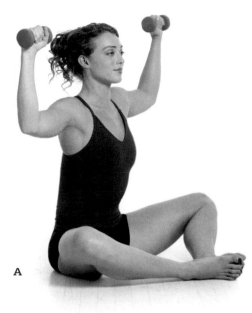

A

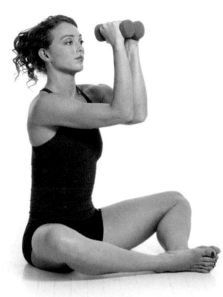

B

Cobbler
with Chest Fly

A From a seated position, bring the soles of your feet together and let your knees fall wide apart. Grab your weights and bring your elbows to shoulder level, with your palms facing front. **B** Take in a deep breath and exhale as you bring your forearms together, elbows touching. Then pull your arms back out to your sides, opening your chest area. Try to keep your elbows in line with your shoulders as you bring your forearms back together in front of you. Let's do this 5 times slowly. This is going to sculpt your back as you are stretching your hips and inner thighs.

mat matters

For an extra challenge, you can do a Mini-Lift when your elbows touch by lifting your arms over your head.

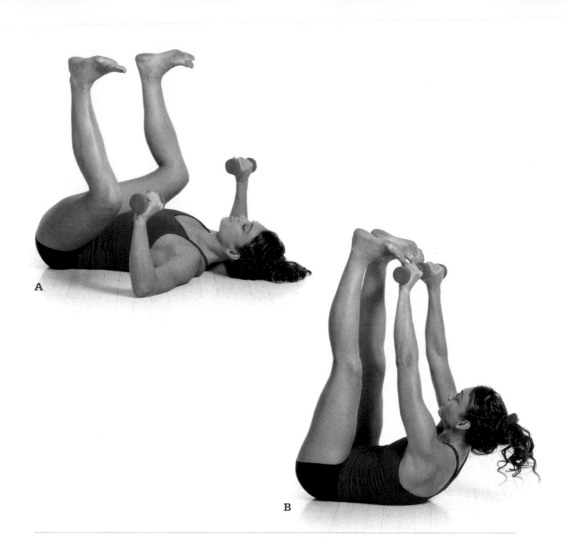

Dead Bug with Chest Press

A Lie down on your back and bring your knees to your chest. Grab your weights, with your elbows bent. **B** Take in a deep breath and exhale as you lift your weights and extend your legs toward the ceiling. Keep your feet flexed. Try to lift your hips and shoulders off the mat as you bring your weights to your toes. Hold for 5 seconds. (Be sure to pause at the top. You'll be able to feel your belly flattening during this one!) Release your knees to the outside of your chest as you lower your weights back down to the mat. Do this 5 times. Once you are finished, place your weights by your side and hug your knees into your chest. Rock side to side, releasing your lower back. From here release, your feet to the floor.

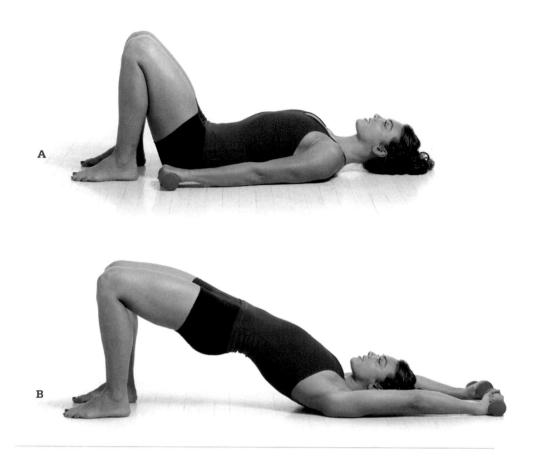

Advanced Bridge with a Lift

Ⓐ Lie down on the floor with your knees bent and your feet hip-distance apart. Reach down with your fingertips to see if you can reach your feet. If not, walk your feet a little closer to your body. Grab your weights and hold them next to your hips, palms facing down. Ⓑ Take in a deep breath and as you exhale, press your weight into your feet to lift your hips while simultaneously bringing your arms over and behind your head. As your hips rise, the backs of your hands should touch the mat or floor. Then bring your weights back down as you lower your hips back to the floor. We are going to do this 5 times. On the last time, take in a deep breath and exhale as you lower your arms and legs to the floor.

Core+ 30-Minute Workout

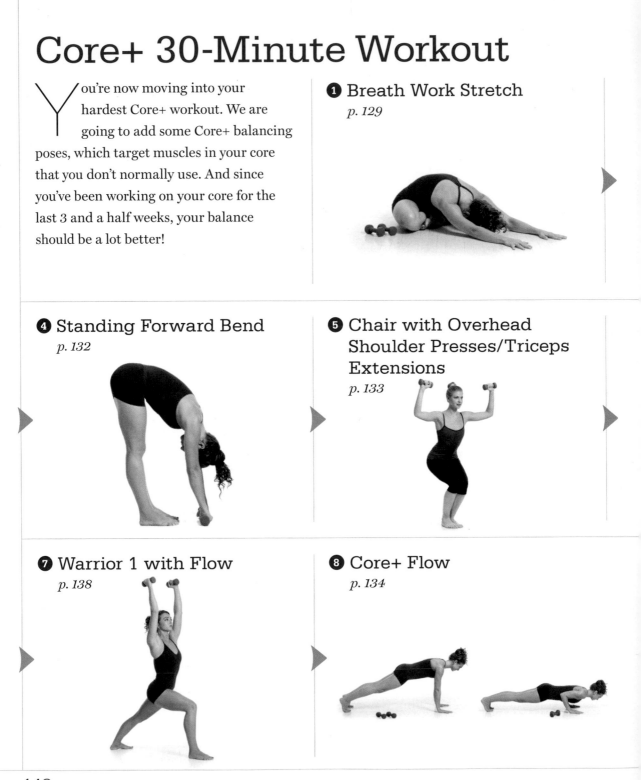

You're now moving into your hardest Core+ workout. We are going to add some Core+ balancing poses, which target muscles in your core that you don't normally use. And since you've been working on your core for the last 3 and a half weeks, your balance should be a lot better!

❶ Breath Work Stretch
p. 129

❹ Standing Forward Bend
p. 132

❺ Chair with Overhead Shoulder Presses/Triceps Extensions
p. 133

❼ Warrior 1 with Flow
p. 138

❽ Core+ Flow
p. 134

② Easy Spinal Twist
p. 89

③ Rock Up and Reach
p. 130

⑥ Core+ Flow (3 times)
p. 134

⑨ Warrior 1 with Flow
p. 138

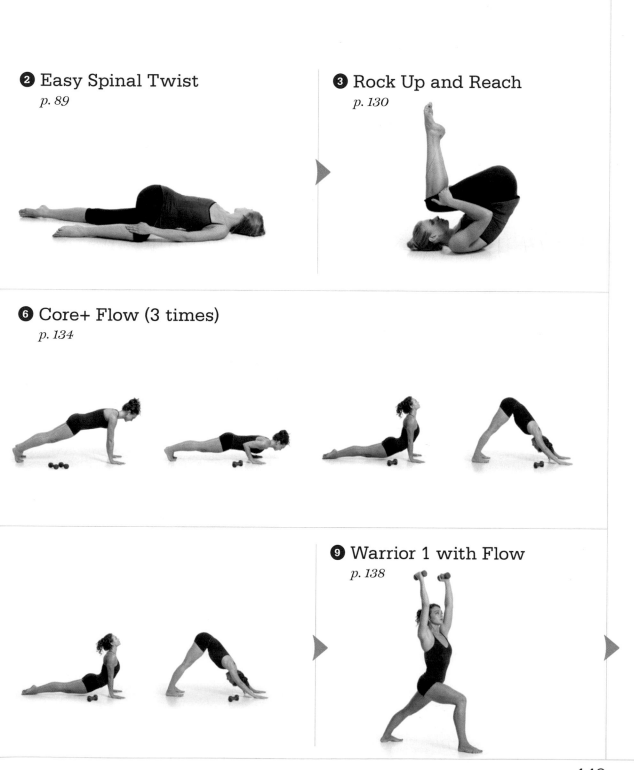

Core+ 30-Minute Workout *(cont.)*

10 Core+ Flow
p. 134

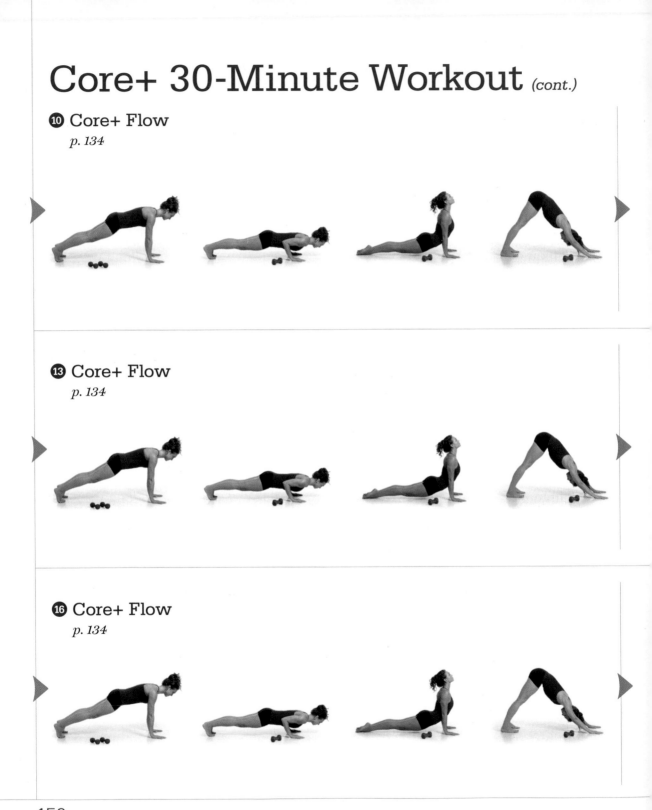

13 Core+ Flow
p. 134

16 Core+ Flow
p. 134

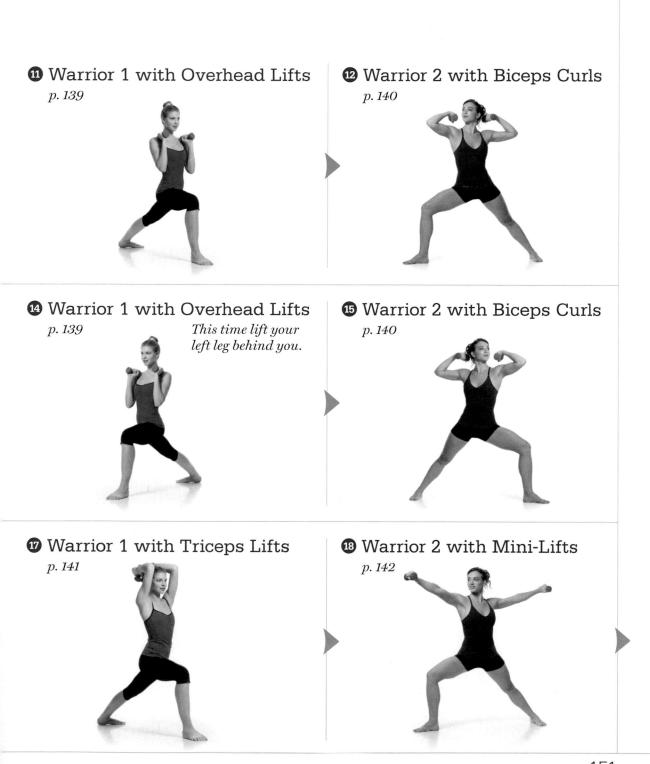

⑪ Warrior 1 with Overhead Lifts
p. 139

⑫ Warrior 2 with Biceps Curls
p. 140

⑭ Warrior 1 with Overhead Lifts
p. 139
This time lift your left leg behind you.

⑮ Warrior 2 with Biceps Curls
p. 140

⑰ Warrior 1 with Triceps Lifts
p. 141

⑱ Warrior 2 with Mini-Lifts
p. 142

Core+ 30-Minute Workout *(cont.)*

19 Side Angle with Lat Rows
p. 143

20 Core+ Flow
p. 134

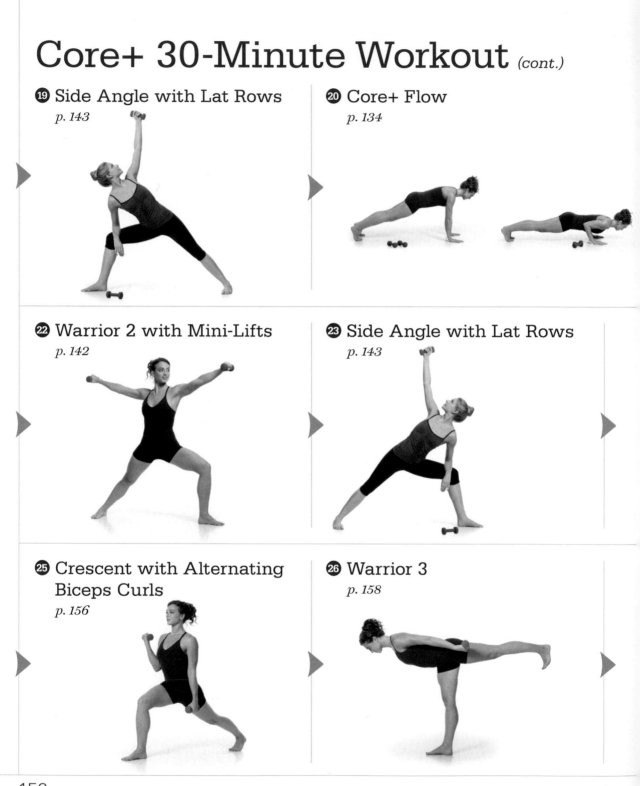

22 Warrior 2 with Mini-Lifts
p. 142

23 Side Angle with Lat Rows
p. 143

25 Crescent with Alternating Biceps Curls
p. 156

26 Warrior 3
p. 158

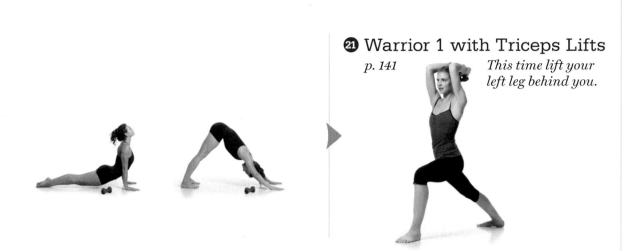

㉑ Warrior 1 with Triceps Lifts
p. 141 *This time lift your left leg behind you.*

㉔ Core+ Flow
p. 134

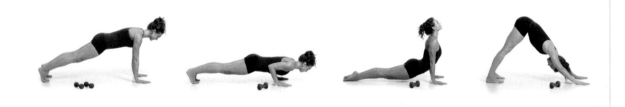

㉗ Core+ Flow
p. 134

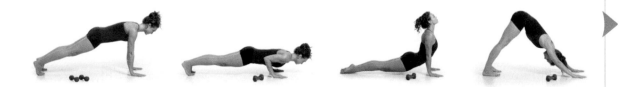

Core+ 30-Minute Workout *(cont.)*

28 Crescent with Alternating Biceps Curls

p. 156

This time lift your left leg behind you.

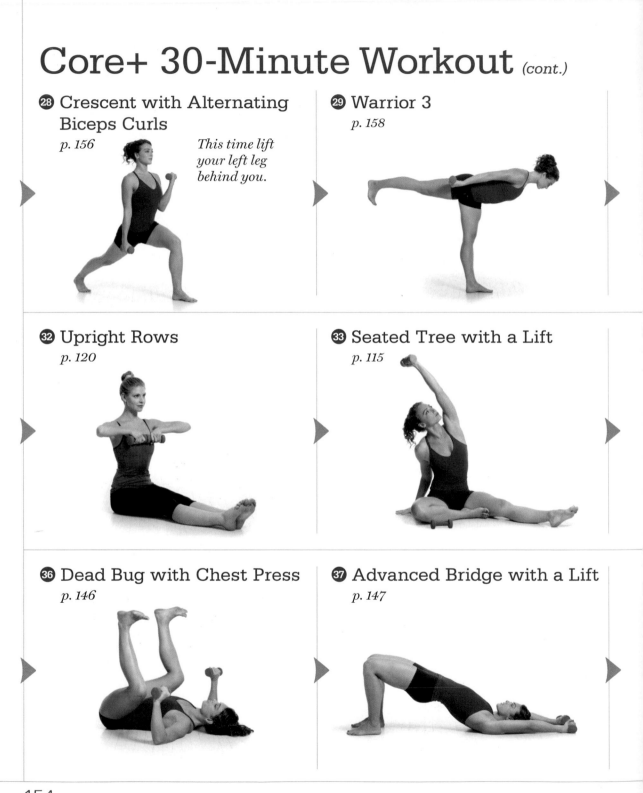

29 Warrior 3

p. 158

32 Upright Rows

p. 120

33 Seated Tree with a Lift

p. 115

36 Dead Bug with Chest Press

p. 146

37 Advanced Bridge with a Lift

p. 147

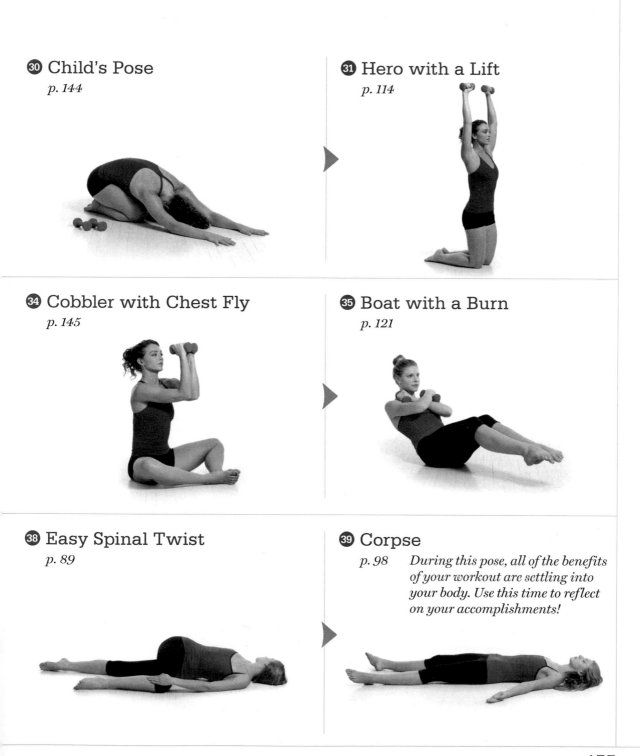

30 Child's Pose
p. 144

31 Hero with a Lift
p. 114

34 Cobbler with Chest Fly
p. 145

35 Boat with a Burn
p. 121

38 Easy Spinal Twist
p. 89

39 Corpse
p. 98   *During this pose, all of the benefits of your workout are settling into your body. Use this time to reflect on your accomplishments!*

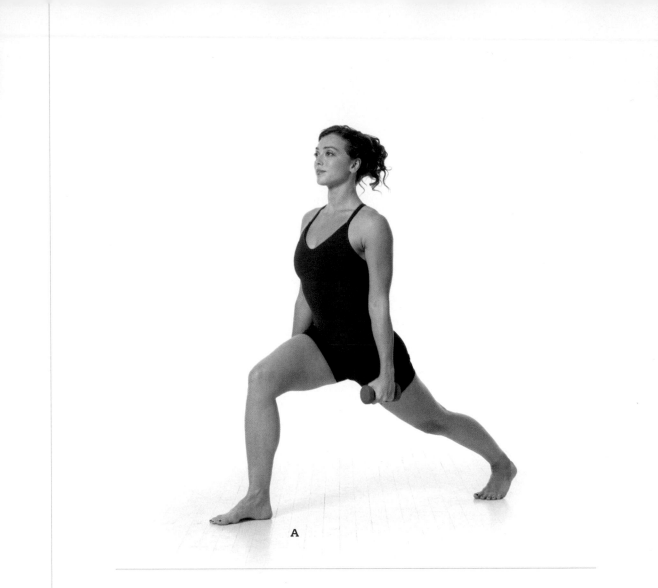

A

Crescent with Alternating Biceps Curls

Starting from Downward Facing Dog, lift your right leg toward the ceiling. Shift your weight onto the ball of your back foot and swing your right leg through your hands. Make sure your back leg is straight and strong. **A** Keeping yourself balanced, grab your weights and let them hang down by your hips. From here we are going to do Alternating Biceps Curls, beginning with your right arm. **B** Slowly bring your right hand up toward your shoulder. **C** As you lower it back down again, raise your left hand. Do this 4 more times.

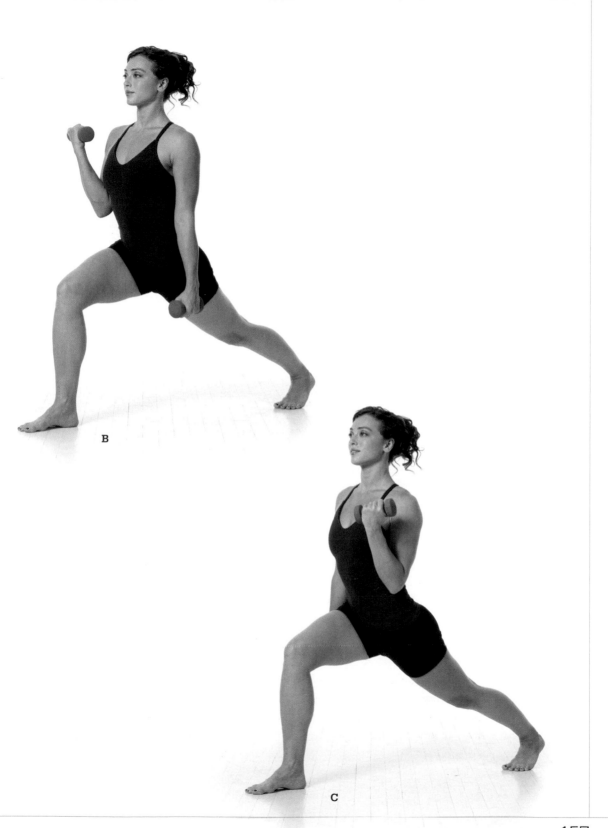

B

C

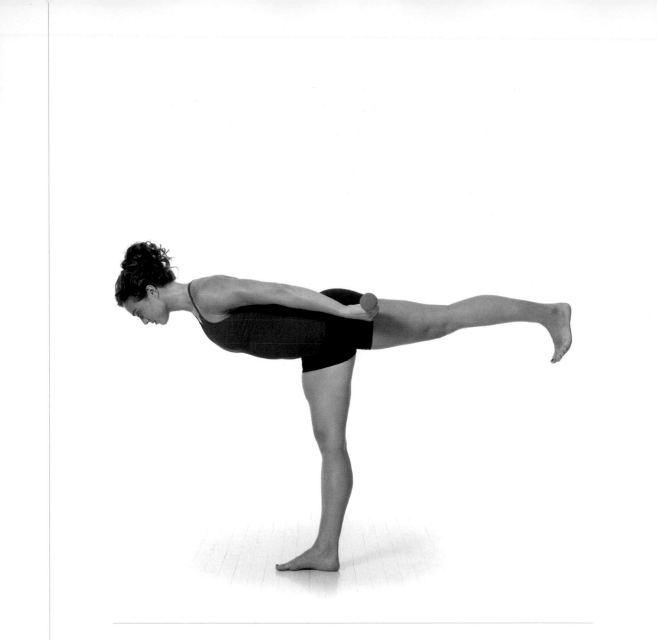

Warrior 3

Starting from Crescent, bring your arms alongside your hips, allowing them to hang by your sides. Slowly shift your weight forward, then straighten your standing leg. Keep your arms next to your hips and raise your back leg to hip level. The goal of this pose is to shape your body to look like the letter T. From here, drop your raised leg down by the other and bend forward at your hips. You can bend your knees to release your lower back.

Wow, you've finished your Flat Belly Yoga! 4-Week Workout! Now it's time to get measured and see how far you've come. Go back to Chapter 5 and pull your measurements from Day 1 of your 4-Day Jump Start. Enter them in the left column below. You probably already know you've lost weight, right? You don't have to weigh yourself to know that your clothes are a lot looser! But just so we can see your progress, hop on your scale now and get out that tape measure to record your new numbers.

Start Date	**End Date**
WEIGHT:	**WEIGHT:**
WAIST: (The most important number!)	**WAIST:** (The most important number!)
CHEST:	**CHEST:**
LEFT BICEP:	**LEFT BICEP:**
RIGHT BICEP:	**RIGHT BICEP:**
HIPS:	**HIPS:**
LEFT THIGH:	**LEFT THIGH:**
RIGHT THIGH:	**RIGHT THIGH:**

Jennifer Bauer

Age: 40

Pounds lost:

17.5

in 32 days

All-over inches lost:

22.75

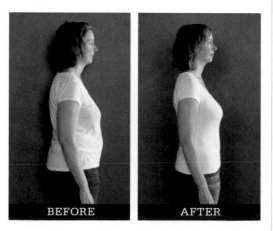

BEFORE   AFTER

"I've had two back surgeries in the last 10 years," says Jennifer Bauer. "Before the second surgery, my doctor tried a round of cortisone that resulted in some really quick weight gain (and excess stomach fat) that I just couldn't seem to lose."

Jennifer, who describes herself as a person in "pretty good shape," had a hard time shedding that stubborn belly fat and was motivated to try something new when she found out about the Flat Belly Yoga! Workout. Determined to stay focused, she even signed up her husband for the program. Together, they followed the workout and the diet, and she began to see results quickly.

"I lost a couple of pounds the first week, but there wasn't really a body shift," she explains. "But after the second week, I really started to notice a difference. I had definitely lost more weight, and my clothes were starting to fit differently."

By the third week, Jennifer's friends and family started to notice a change and asked if she was dieting. And by Week 4, the change was obvious: Jennifer had dropped an astonishing two sizes.

"By the last week, I had a closet full of clothes that no longer fit. I had to use a belt to hold up my pants," she says. "I had a work event that week, and my colleague actually noted that she could tell how much slimmer I was. It was really that noticeable. I could even fit into jeans that I hadn't worn in over 5 years!"

Jennifer credits her success to having a support system and making the most out of her workout time. "I really enjoyed sharing this experience with my husband. We worked together to make sure we were both making time for exercise." And on days when it was particularly hard for her to find the time to work out, she combined her Heart Walk with a stroller walk so that she could spend some extra time with her child. This provided more time in the evening for her Core+ Yoga workout.

Though she had been practicing yoga for a few years, the 40-year-old says incorporating weights increased her strength quickly. "I felt stronger, and that was motivating. I was pretty familiar with the yoga poses, but I couldn't use weights the entire time at the beginning. Now, I use the 3-pound weights with no problem. And for some of the poses, I even use 5-pound weights," she exclaims. "Before, I did not exercise every day. But this program really helped me see the importance of making time to exercise 6 days a week. Now it's a necessity—not just a maybe."

Because Jennifer enjoyed the program so much, she plans to continue her daily Core+ Yoga workout and Heart Walk. "It was an amazing feeling to complete the program. I was surprised at how fast the time went. And I feel much better about my belly now. I have already proven to myself that I can make time every day to exercise. There is no reason to stop now. 99

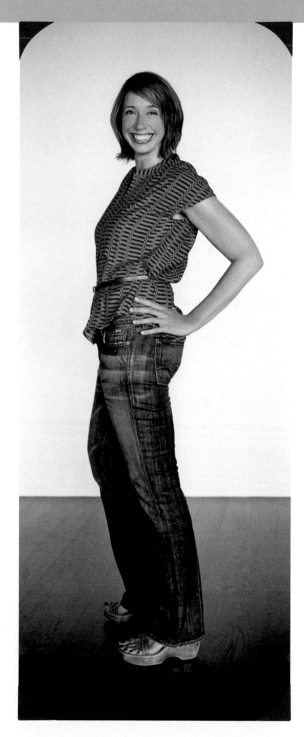

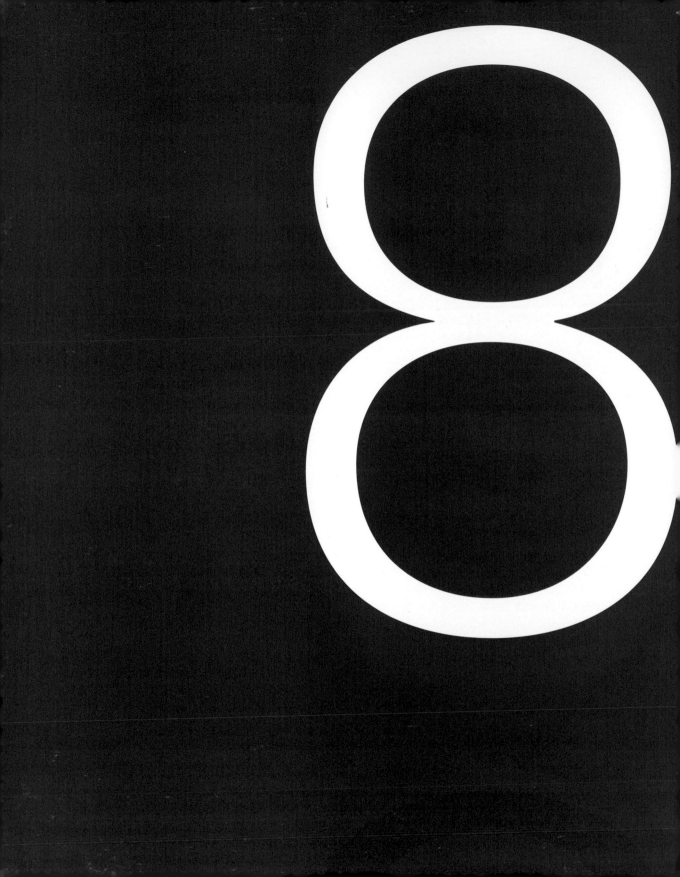

CREATING TIME FOR WORKOUTS

I'd work out. *I would, I really would! But . . . I don't have the time.* There. I said it for you, so you don't have to. I know you were thinking it. We *all* think it. And guess what? We all reinforce it for each other, too. When you look around, it's easy to let yourself believe that no one has enough time for anything anymore. Well, except for sitting at the computer, whether you're working, perusing social media, or watching YouTube videos. Right? "Not enough time" is, in fact, the number one reason most of us give for why we don't work out.

It's Just Sitting Around—Or Is It?

According to the American Time Use Survey, the average American now sits more than they sleep—9.3 hours per day of sitting versus 7.7 hours of sleep.[1] And you know what? It's not good for us. Too much sitting contributes to obesity, diabetes, cancer, and simply dying earlier than we otherwise would if we remembered to get up and move around.

To reduce your cancer risk, the American Institute for Cancer Research is urging Americans to add mini-breaks from sitting to a daily regimen of getting at least 30 minutes a day of moderate-to-vigorous exercise. And that's exactly what I'm asking you to do.

"If you reduce sitting by 5 minutes an hour, at the end of a long day, you've shaved an hour off your total sitting time," says Alpa V. Patel, PhD, an epidemiologist at the American Cancer Society. That advice also applies to "active couch potatoes," who hit the gym or take that daily brisk walk, as some research indicates daily exercise is not enough to protect against the harmful effects of prolonged sitting.[2]

According to one study in the American Society for Clinical Nutrition, even *fidgeting* can combat the negative effects of too much sitting.[3] Study subjects who had a habit of fidgeting burned significantly more calories and became much less obese than those who simply sat still. So we're going to take some of that harmful sitting time and put it right into your Flat Belly Yoga! Workout routine. Whether you're sitting in traffic, at your desk, at your home computer, or around the house talking on the phone, by turning your sitting time into exercise time, you're going to kill two birds with one stone: You'll reduce the harmful impact from all that sitting while successfully accomplishing the workouts that your negative, nagging "I don't have the time" voice often prevents.

You've Come to the Right Place

Flat Belly Yoga! already accounts for time constraints by including efficient (read: speedy) Core+ Yoga sessions. You might have looked through Chapter 7 and thought, "How am I going to fit all of that yoga into my busy day?" Well, I have news for you: While most yoga classes are 90 minutes long, with an occasional few lasting only 1 hour, the Core+ workouts are all 30 minutes or less. By picking up this book, you've already given yourself an advantage that you wouldn't have if you had signed up for a class at a studio.

The simplicity of the Heart Walk routines is another time advantage because you can be creative about when and where you get your cardio exercise. Let's look for ways to fit in some daily cardio exercises that work for you. I bet we can come up with a few ideas that are convenient—even for your busy schedule.

I know it's very likely that your first 4 days during the Jump Start will present you with some obstacles to meeting your workout commitments. My goal here is to get you to think of working out as a necessary part of every day, not as a luxury that you can fit in when you have the time and the energy. It should be as automatic as brushing your teeth. (But much more fun!)

My belief is that these tips and tricks will be a lot of help during the 4-Day Jump Start and during the first half of the 4-Week Workout. But I also think that you will find yourself turning back to this chapter less and less as your workouts go on. Why? Because as you progress with your workouts, you're going to automatically come up with tips and tricks of your own to defend your workout time or sneak it into your busiest days. But until then, let's learn how to take back those lost moments during the day and use them for your workouts!

Take Back Your Time

Some days you just can't find the time for a full workout. The most important thing to do when that happens is *not give up*. I'm going to encourage you to find a way to make it happen.

Adding just a few minutes of physical exercise a day has huge benefits on your health, gives you energy, and perks up your mood. In fact, one study found that if inactive people increased their physical activity by just 15 minutes per day, they could reduce their risk of premature death by 14 percent and increase their life expectancy by 3 years.[4]

So now are you thinking of the time issue as a puzzle worth solving? I hope so. But that still leaves one question: Where can you find the time?

Let's Get You Moving

The following pages feature a number of quick Flat Belly Yoga! Workout tips. Some of them will work anywhere, anytime. Others are specific to your circumstances. As you look through them and think about which ones best fit into your life and routines, keep in mind that doing even a little bit of exercise—even if it's just 5 to 10 minutes at a time—will make a big difference in your day. And they will move you forward on your daily quest for a flatter belly! Here are some tips to help you find ways to incorporate workouts into your busy days.

Parking Lot Cardio. Here's the scenario: You're circling the parking lot, looking for the close-to-the-door space that will allow you to get in and out. If you can just get your groceries and get home, maybe you'll have time for a walk. You have the perfect spot in sight until someone swoops in and takes it from you! Instead of trying to find the perfect spot, head for the farthest, emptiest corner of the lot and walk the extra distance. And if you only have one or two bags of groceries, leave the cart at the entrance of the store and walk all the way around the parking lot on your way back to the car— now you're walking with weights! Imagine the benefits: You're getting in your workout while also relieving the stress of trying to make it home in time to fit in your routine.

Change Your Station. Take the bus or the subway? Unless you live right next door, you probably already get a little exercise walking to and from the station. Now it's time to give yourself a little more. Try getting off one stop early and walking the rest of the way to your house or your workplace. Do that for a week. Next week, try two stops and incorporate some interval training. It may take a little longer to get home in the evenings, but then all of your time at home can be spent on other activities.

Make Things Inconvenient. Need to borrow a cup of sugar from your neighbor? Why don't you walk all the way to the store? Or how about that prescription you need to pick up from the pharmacy? Walk there.

Perhaps you need to drop off that blouse at the dry cleaner's. Got a pair of slacks, too? If you "forget" them at home the first time, then you have a great reason to turn right around and walk back! If it's too far to walk the whole distance, drive half of the way and walk the rest. Have you ever seen a nice, shaded parking space on a side street, but it was just a little too far from your destination? Now you have a reason to go ahead and take it!

Take a Lap. This terrific suggestion was supplied by one of my students at my studio in Venice, California. She mentioned that her schedule didn't really allow her to get anything done while her son was at soccer practice. At first, she would drive him to practice, then drive home and get frustrated with herself because she couldn't accomplish anything in the small amount of time she had between dropping him off and turning back around to pick him up. Then she decided to just stay at the field and relax. But instead of relaxing, she found herself thinking of all the items on her to-do list. Finally she realized that if her son was going to run around the whole time, she should, too! So now she no longer just sits around watching her son play soccer. (It's fun on game day, but let's face it—as wonderful as kids are, you don't have to watch every move at every practice.) Instead, she takes a lap (or two) around the field.

AROUND THE WORLD IN 80 WORKOUTS

Travel is one of the easiest ways to get thrown off of a workout routine. But all the workouts in *Flat Belly Yoga!* are portable, so there's no reason to miss one—ever:

- Buy a slightly larger bag if you need extra room to pack your walking shoes and workout clothes. And remember, you don't have to drop your dollars on piles and piles of gear. The carpet in your hotel room is all the mat you'll need.

- If you're on a business trip and your colleague says, "I guess I'm going to have to skip my workout because this hotel doesn't have a fitness center," you're not allowed to piggyback on his or her excuse. Your body *is* your fitness center! Even if you're traveling to Alaska in January, you can still do a Heart Walk in the halls and stairwells of your hotel. The people looking at you don't think you're strange. They know exactly what you're doing. And they envy you!

- Ask hotel staff to recommend a nearby park where can you can do your Heart Walk and learn a little bit more about your current location. There may be an architecturally interesting neighborhood or a fun downtown district that will make for a nice place to change up your routine. Stop thinking of your travel as an obstacle to your routine and start thinking of it as an opportunity to add some spice to it.

And keep this in mind: If jet lag or an extremely busy schedule leaves you too tired to function, make your workout a little shorter or lighter. It's okay to adjust your workout every now and then—as long as you get back on track when your energy returns.

USE YOUR LUNCH BREAKS

I'm not going to tell you to eat on the run because sticking to regular eating patterns is a helpful tactic in the battle of the bulge.[5] Some researchers also think that the very act of eating irregularly may contribute to obesity. Neurological evidence indicates that the brain's biological clock—the pacemaker that controls numerous other daily rhythms in our bodies—may also help to regulate hunger and satiety signals. Ideally, these signals should keep our weight steady and prompt us to eat when our body fat falls below a certain level. They should also tell us when we feel satiated and should stop eating. Close connections between the brain's pacemaker and the appetite control center in the hypothalamus suggest that hunger and satiety are affected by temporal cues. And irregular eating patterns may disrupt the effectiveness of these cues in a way that promotes obesity.

Keep one thing in mind: Eating in transit may save you some time, but it's not in the best interest of your long-term health and victory over belly fat. So why not try to pack a lunch a few times each week? Instead of going out to eat with your colleagues or stopping at a restaurant for a lunch break, take a Heart Walk. (Invite your colleagues and friends!) Then, when you get back to work, eat your lunch there.

FIND EXTRA TIME

Put on your detective hat and do a little sleuthing to figure out where you spend your extra time. "But Kimberly, I don't have any extra time," you may say. A likely alibi. We're assigning a top-notch private eye to the case: your journal. This is why it's so great to keep a journal. (I believe that keeping a daily record of your exercise routines, goals, and accomplishments is one of the most important parts of achieving what you want with exercise, as you'll see in Chapter 9 on page 177.)

As you look around, you might actually find some "time-sucks" that you weren't previously aware of:

- Maybe you'll discover that you spend way too much time on the phone with your best friend. I know she's funny and interesting, but your health is more important! If you can't seem to tear yourself away, hook up a wired headset or Bluetooth, to your cell and talk to your funny friend while you are walking. That's 30 minutes that you would have spent sitting in your living room on the phone, and now you have completed your Heart Walk! (Also, now is not the time to tell your friend that she doesn't ask you enough questions about your life. The more she talks about herself without permitting interruptions, the more you'll be able to get into the interval training.)

- Do you use social media? In the course of human history, there has been no greater time-suck invented than social media! With the addition of the streaming sidebar updates, you can get caught up in every minute of your friends' friends' lives. Step away from your computer and spend some time thinking about you. Ask yourself how much you care where your friend Tim's uncle had coffee. Not much, right?

- With your computer in general, you can find software that helps you show how much time you spend using each aspect—surfing the Web, sending e-mail, and even working in applications such as your word processor, spreadsheets, and PowerPoint. RescueTime (www.rescuetime.com) is the best-known free computer-usage tracker, but a quick search will turn up others. I've never used this program because I already know what takes up the most of my time: e-mails. Time Out (www.dejal.com) is a nice application you can program to force you to take breaks—it actually locks you out of your computer for a set amount of time. Why not program it to kick you off the computer for 15 minutes every 2 hours, and then see how far you can walk during your regularly scheduled break? This seems a little drastic, but you might want to try it if you're having trouble breaking away from your screen.

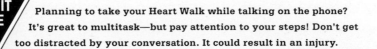

PLAY IT SAFE Planning to take your Heart Walk while talking on the phone? It's great to multitask—but pay attention to your steps! Don't get too distracted by your conversation. It could result in an injury.

THE REVERSE SNOOZE ALARM

It's simple: Wake up a little earlier. Sleep is very important, but studies show that working out can actually help you get *more* sleep.

You'll sleep more deeply if you exercise regularly. And you don't have to be a star athlete to reap the benefits—as little as 20 to 30 minutes of daily activity can make a difference. Also, you don't have to complete all 30 minutes at once. You can break it up into 5 minutes here or 10 minutes there and still get the benefits. Try a brisk walk, a bicycle ride, or even gardening or housework.

It's not necessarily the case that you should exercise right before you go to sleep—for some people, that revs up their engines and makes it harder for them to fall asleep. The important thing is that if you go to bed earlier and get up 30 minutes earlier, you can then use that time to do your workout. And it's much better than a cup of coffee!

WALK, DON'T RERUN

Isn't it fascinating how much time we spend in front of the TV? I have to admit, I love to watch a little *People's Court* (who doesn't love Judge Marilyn Milian?) and maybe an occasional episode of *Law & Order*. (Don't ask me why legal or cop shows calm me down.) But an episode fills a half hour. There's your missing workout time.

As I've said before, I'm not going to ask you to give up your favorite shows. So I'll give you another option: Do your Core+ Yoga workout while you are watching your favorite TV show. Now you can take your time, stretch it out, and work extra hard during the commercial breaks.

REFRAME THE PICTURE OF WORKING OUT

Reframing is a term that politicians use when they talk about changing negative associations into positive ones. If they can do it when they talk to their voters about taxes and spending, you can do it when you talk to yourself about exercise.

Studies have demonstrated that leading individuals to mentally reframe the time required for an exercise program (e.g., 2 hours per week) in terms of the equivalent daily amount (e.g., 17 minutes per day) reduced the perceived time commitment and increased people's willingness to try the program.[6]

STEP AWAY FROM YES

Think about it: How much activity is in your life because it's convenient for other people? Do you find yourself picking up a friend's dry cleaning or listening to them gab away on the phone for hours? Just say no! I know this is hard, especially for women. But your friends will love you even if you're not doing things they "need" you to do. And if they don't, they're not your friends. Think about it: Do you really need to do everything people ask you to? Say it loud, say it proud, say *no*!

CANCELLATIONS WILL BE BILLED AS A FULL VISIT

Schedule your workout exactly like it was a doctor's appointment. This doesn't give you extra time—it places a value on your time. And why shouldn't you value your time as much as your doctor values her time? This will help make you be more accountable to yourself. You wouldn't cancel on your doctor, would you? Treat your workouts like an appointment with your health.

We Have the Technology

Scientists don't really believe that we use only 10 percent of our brains. That's a myth. However, it could be argued that we use only 10 percent of our smartphones. There are terrific apps to help you exercise, but one of the simplest ones that you don't even have to download is . . . *the calendar*. What's the point of having a "smart"phone if you're going to let it play dumb about you missing your workouts? Use the calendar app to add reminders to your phone, and make sure the reminders are *loud*.

I use calendar reminders for everything and even have little beeps going off to remind me to take my vitamins. Don't just add a general reminder to work out—add one for your Heart Walk and another one for your Core+ Yoga routine. Setting specific reminders will come in handy, especially when you first begin the 4-Day Jump Start. Remember, the goal is to get you into a workout routine and make it a habit every day. So here's one extra tip for using your technology: I don't click off the reminder until I do whatever it's reminding me to do. It keeps me honest and accountable—and it gives me a sense of accomplishment.

Getting to the Core+ of the Matter

Most of the tips I've provided are useful for finding time to incorporate or schedule your Heart Walks. But it's also important to find time for your Core+ Yoga routines. Here are a few ways to fit in your Core+ exercises when you're out and about.

Curl it up. Carry your groceries to the edge of the parking lot—or, even better, all the way home. Now add a few biceps curls with your heavy bags in your hands. That's right, the potato has now become an official part of the Flat Belly Yoga! Workout!

Stair-ing contest. Make sure you're standing up straight as you walk up stairs. (This will automatically engage your core.) All it takes is directed focus for you to derive an exercise benefit.

Plank you very much. Once you've already made the time for your Core+ workouts, add a few extra seconds to your hold in the Plank Pose (page 134). It may look pretty simple, but it's really one of the best poses you can do to increase your core strength. So take your time and hold this for as long as you can.

Strike a pose. While you're on the phone, take a lesson from Madonna's song "Vogue" and "strike a pose!" Even holding just a couple of poses during a conversation will add valuable workout minutes that you wouldn't have gotten otherwise. Plank isn't very easy (unless you're on speakerphone and your best friend is still talking about herself). But there are a number of other poses you can work into a phone conversation, especially if you have a headset. So now is the time to get creative!

The Chair Pose (page 91) is a good place to start. If you're holding on to the phone, keep one arm straight out in front for balance. Warrior 1 (page 92) works, too (although you might want to switch your arms if you're going into this pose directly after the Chair Pose). You can also try the Hero Pose found on page 93. You can talk through most of the poses that make up your Core+ workouts—just don't try anything that requires a lot of balance or concentration so that you don't fall and injure yourself. (Don't try Bridge on the phone. It's just not a good idea.)

No Time Like the Present

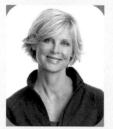

I've never been the kind of person who likes a lot of downtime. I'd rather be climbing a mountain than napping on the couch or switching channels in front of the TV.

Truth is, these days few of us have much leisure time even if that's the thing we crave the most. Our lives are packed with activities—work, commuting, shopping, cleaning, family obligations, and so on.

So where does exercise fit into the picture?

For me, exercise is always the last thing that gets cut from my schedule, never the first. I think of it like eating or getting dressed or going to work—it's a required course, not an elective.

This might sound funny, but if I get a call right before a workout, I tell the person on the other line that I am stepping into a meeting and that I'll call them back in an hour. I hear my students do the same thing all the time. We do it because it works, but also because it's a way of declaring to ourselves that our fitness is as important as anything else. You can't think of it as a luxury or something you squeeze in around other things.

If you are someone who has a hard time finding the time to work out, you might want to try making a list of the things that are most important to you. Now exercise might not be on the list, but I'm pretty sure health, looking good, and feeling good will be. And if they're not, that raises some pretty serious questions, don't you think?

If you're still fixated on the time issue, here's what I suggest: Calculate how much time you'll spend exercising over the next 20 years if you work out 6 days a week for 40 minutes a day. Then compare that to what the experts tell us about how much longer you'll live—and how much better the quality of your life will be—as a result of that time spent getting in shape. If you're not a math whiz, I'll save you the effort: Committing to a regular exercise routine like the Flat Belly Yoga! Workout will net you significant time over the course of your life—time that you'll enjoy far more than you would have if you never got off the couch.

So no matter how busy you are, make room for exercise—it will pay off in the ways that really matter.

A FLAT BELLY YOGA SUCCESS STORY

Paul Neely

Age: 47

Pounds lost:
10.5
in 32 days

All-over inches lost:
15.5

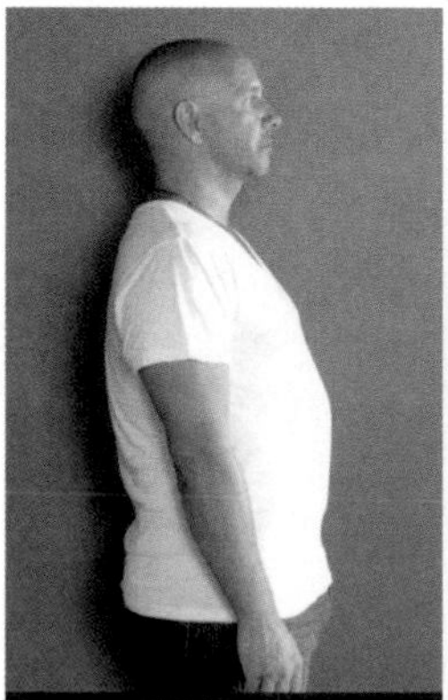

BEFORE

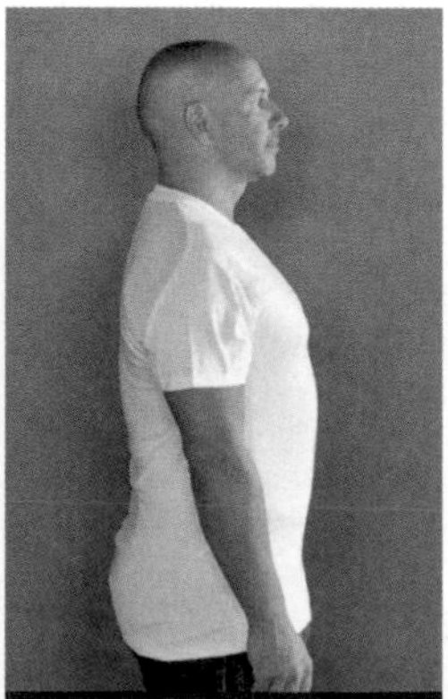

AFTER

"I used to be able to drop any weight that I had gained within 3 weeks, but suddenly it seemed like nothing worked," says Paul Neely. "I have been struggling with weight gain since 2008, and the battle was more difficult than ever before."

Realizing it was time for a change, Paul decided to try the Flat Belly Yoga! Workout. Having practiced yoga before, he knew he would enjoy a yoga-based routine and make the time for it, which was important because of his hectic work schedule. "I really felt that I was at the point where something needed to change. But I knew that trying to fit a plan into my schedule while working and traveling would be difficult."

Soon after beginning the program, Paul was sent to the Dominican Republic of the Congo, a country located in central Africa, for work. It was during this time that he began struggling with making time for his workouts.

"While there, my biggest challenge was finding the correct time and space to do my workouts. In the larger city, Kinshasa, I had a standardized western-type hotel room, which made it much simpler. I moved the furniture around and woke up early to do my workout. That was when I had the highest level of energy and peace of mind."

But Paul's schedule changed constantly during his trip. And when it came time to travel again to another location with his coworkers, finding the time to complete his workout became an even greater challenge than before. "Not only were the hotel rooms and makeshift overnight places challenging for me, but the constant companionship of my colleagues, who, like myself, were confronted with ongoing changes, also proved difficult. Breakfasts, lunches, dinners, and travel time were almost always spent together as a group," he says. "One of my ways of dealing with all of this was to actually sense a window or sudden down time at any given moment in the day and do my Core+ Yoga workout."

Paul realized that once he adjusted to the idea of working out at a moment's notice, things became easier for him. "Usually once I was into the workout by approximately 10 minutes, all was forgotten and I could find my flow and connect with my workout." To incorporate his Heart Walks, Paul took advantage of his surroundings, walking around the villages or towns at least once each day.

By the end of his trip, Paul had lost 3.5 inches from his belly and over 10 pounds, and he gained a renewed love of exercise. "I forgot how great it feels to take time out for yourself and exercise. And it's easy—I can work up a sweat from something that isn't too difficult," he says. "It felt good to complete the Flat Belly Yoga! program, but I want to keep going. I don't feel like anything is 'over' at the moment—just a good start to maintaining a workout, because it finally seems doable. ❞

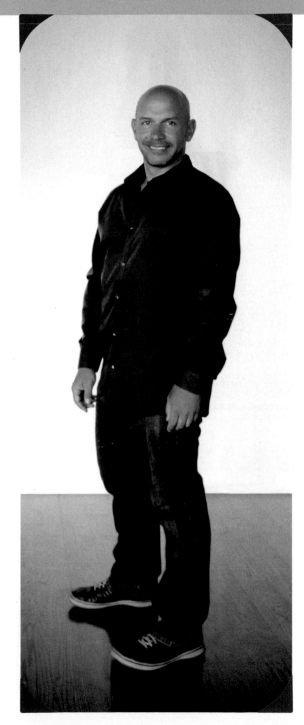

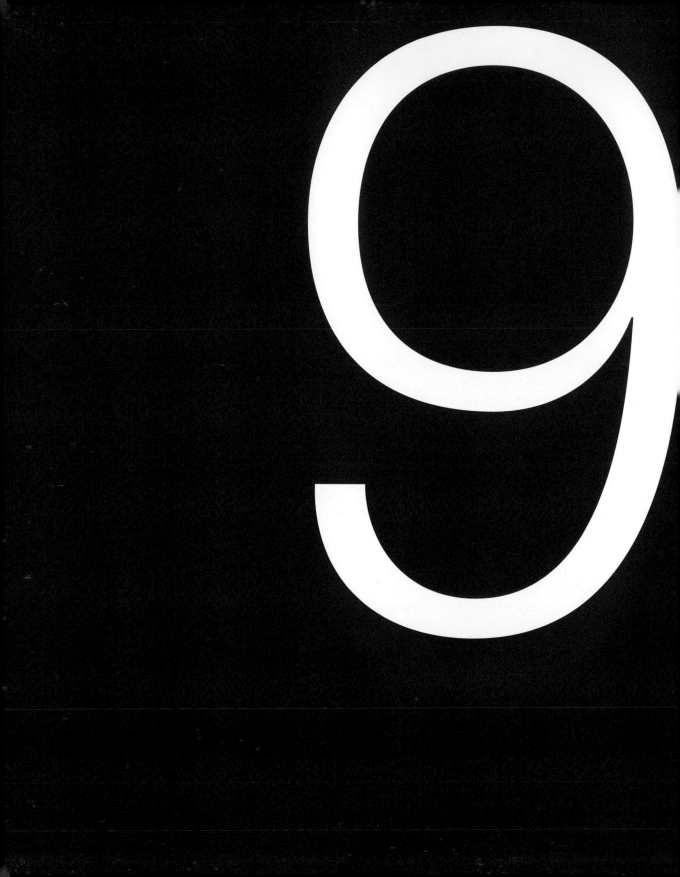

THE FLAT BELLY YOGA! JOURNAL

Most of us have heard how effective keeping a journal can be for dieting or establishing new eating habits. But did you know that journaling can be just as effective for helping you establish and stick with a new workout routine? Learning to recognize and respect your efforts can really help you achieve your goals, and keeping your Flat Belly Yoga! Journal will help you do just that.

Write Yourself Healthy

Believe it or not, there is increasing evidence to support the notion that simply writing down your experiences in a journal can have a positive impact your physical well-being.

In one study, researchers at Stony Brook University in New York asked people with asthma or rheumatoid arthritis to journal about the most stressful experiences of their lives. All they had to do was write for 20 minutes a day, for 3 days. Just that alone—no more—made asthma patients breathe better, while the arthritis patients had less pain and swelling. And the patients' results lasted for at least 4 months.[1]

How can this be? Remember when we talked about stress and how it makes your sympathetic nervous system fight-or-flight response kick in? And how being under chronic stress makes your body release more of certain hormones, like adrenaline and cortisol? Those hormones have real, lasting effects on your body. De-stressing, however you do it, makes those hormones drop, and that can improve your health in a number of ways.

CHANGE YOUR BRAIN

So how can a journal make you de-stress? After all, if the participants in the study mentioned above had to focus on their most stressful memories, wouldn't that create more stress?

Scientists have been working on figuring this out since the 1980s, when therapists started to use journaling as a therapy for people dealing with major traumas. At first, they thought it was just about releasing pent-up stress and how good that made people feel. But eventually they came to believe that journaling actually changes the way your brain works and can even make it easier to stay focused on a simple task.

THE NEGATIVE LOOP

Sometimes working out can bring out negative emotions. Why is this? Well, whenever we work out, we can't avoid thinking about our bodies. We notice all the things that we're unhappy about and the negative self-talk loop starts to play.

Or maybe you're doing a certain yoga pose and a muscle that has been tense for years start to relax. This is no ordinary stretch and release. All of a sudden, you might find yourself overwhelmed with emotion. This kind of thing happens all the time in yoga. In the classroom, yoga teachers even know to expect it. Poses that tap into tension in the back, such as the Easy Spinal Twist, seem to be the most likely to prompt emotional releases during yoga sessions. Frustration and anger could manifest in spinal tension. Heartbreak and depression could linger in the chest. And emotional pain from the past could lie dormant in the hip flexors.

Unfortunately, this kind of thing can be a real block to your workout success. Your brain—which isn't stupid—starts to associate working out with feeling bad about yourself. And why would you want to work out if it makes you feel bad? So you find excuses to skip your workout.

BREAKING THE NEGATIVE LOOP

Instead of letting your negative thoughts keep you away from your workouts, I want you to write them down. Simply admitting that you had that negative thought makes it less powerful. Then I want you to change it around to a positive thought and repeat it 10 times. That's how you'll break the association between working out and negative thoughts.

In fact, keep track of *all* the stressors you run into—the things in your life that cause you stress. Writing them down will take away their power, and working out will help you change what they're doing to your body. Remember this from Chapter 4: There is a real connection between stress and gaining weight—especially belly fat. Taking away the power of your stressors by writing about them doesn't just make you happier: It's another path to getting that flat belly you've always desired.

REINFORCING THE POSITIVE

Let's not get too focused on the negative thoughts you may encounter. Working out also makes you feel *good*. It releases endorphins, which are like the brain's natural, healthy version of a mood-altering substance. You're working on your goals and you have the right to be proud of that. You're burning off your stress *and* your belly fat. Writing it down confirms that what you're doing is good, and it keeps you committed to achieving your goal.

Understanding that there is a mind-body connection—or for our purposes, a mind-belly connection—will help you stay motivated. You might find that as you start the Flat Belly Yoga! program, your energy level rises. You might get up *wanting* to work out!

mat motivation
The Write Stuff

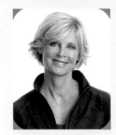

Writing does not come naturally to a lot of people, especially when they have to write about themselves. But I have to say that it can be a very empowering exercise. It helps you gather your thoughts and is a great way to list your goals—giving you a platform to focus on achieving them by making yourself accountable.

My approach is to write down what I call "empowering questions" tied to certain goals I want to accomplish in a certain period of time, like, "What can I do today to make this happen?" I get up very early in the morning and it's one of the first things I do every day. I make myself do five things every day to help me achieve the goal I am focusing on at that time.

Here's an example: I have been working with a well-known credit card company for some time now and had done a few online commercials with them. I wanted to take that relationship to the next level in order to increase the promotion for YAS. Now, my goals can be a bit lofty, but why not aim high? So, I decided that I wanted to be in one of their ads, which are based on small businesses. I wrote it down in my journal as one of my top goals and every day I focused on what I could do to bring myself closer to my goal. To make a very long story short, the company contacted me and asked if I would like to be featured in their next national ad campaign.

Deciding to take control of your health and body is a big goal—an important one—and requires focus time equal to work and family commitments. Write down your goals every day and create a plan to see them through. You might be surprised to see what happens when you stick with it.

BRAINWASH YOURSELF

Scientist after scientist has confirmed that when people write things down, they start to believe what they write. (It's a variation on an old theme that constantly comes back in self-improvement. I bet that once or twice, you've heard someone say, "Fake it till ya make it!")

And a study conducted at Dominican University in River Forest, Illinois, showed that simply keeping a written record of your goals can help you accomplish them. The participants who wrote down their goals accomplished significantly more than those who didn't keep a record their goals.

You can do the same thing for yourself. Set your goals. Write them down. You will believe in them more and you will achieve them. In fact, you can start each workout by writing down your motivation for doing the exercise at hand. Then write down your goal for the end of each workout.

How Am I Doing?

Keeping your Flat Belly Yoga! Journal won't just keep you motivated and help you manage your stress. It will also show you what works for you and what doesn't. And tracking your workouts in your journal will help you stay accountable to yourself.

Get in the habit of writing down the time of day, what you did, and how you felt during your workouts. By doing this every day, you will start to get to know your body. You might find out that you like to work out in the morning. Maybe working out peps you up, giving you the energy you need to attack the day. Or maybe working out relaxes you and helps you burn off stress from a hard day at the office. If that's the case, you should probably exercise in the evening.

I also want you to notice the reasons you haven't worked out in the past. One common excuse is simply not having enough time in a day to fit in a workout. Another excuse: "I'm too tired."

If your excuse is "I don't have the time," use your journal to figure out where you're spending your time. I bet you can uncover a way to make the time. Try watching 5 minutes less of TV. Perhaps you could even record your favorite programs and watch them after you finish your workout or journal entry. Or if you

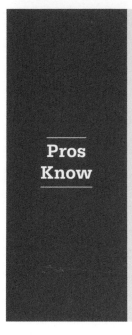

Lots of professional athletes know the power of keeping a journal.

A journal provides an athlete with a place to set goals, reflect, grapple with issues, keep track of training ideas, and record results, as well as serve as a personal diary. Athletes like Serena Williams use their journals for motivation and gaining focus.

Red Sox pitching ace Curt Schilling could be seen on the bench between innings writing notes on the pitches he delivered to certain players during particular situations. Schilling used a journal as a workbook and focused on the technical aspects of his sport.

In England, 16-year-old soccer players who become apprentices to professional teams are required to keep a journal about training sessions, games, diet, etc.

are about to get online, write in your journal before you open up that laptop. You can get on social media or check your email and all of a sudden you've lost a whole hour. Just find a comfortable, private space and write in your journal for 5 minutes. *Then* spend an hour online.

If your excuse is "I'm too tired," use your journal to help you figure out when you have the most energy so that you can work out when you aren't tired. Whatever your excuse, using the Flat Belly Yoga! Journal will help you learn more about yourself and your habits.

KNOW YOUR BODY

Use your journal to keep track of your progress over the next 32 days. How far did you walk today and for how many minutes? If you took three 10-minute breaks during the day to walk, keeping track of the total time you walked in your journal will show you that it really does add up. Which Core+ workout routine did you complete? Was one side of your body stronger than the other? Is it getting easier to hold the weights? How's your form? Keeping track of how your body handles the poses will show you that you really are getting stronger and more balanced.

When you got up from Corpse Pose today, did you feel calmer than you did yesterday, or even a week ago? Keeping track of how your workouts make you feel will let you know you're getting those endorphins we talked about.

COMMIT!

I want you to commit to your workout, commit to getting healthy, and commit to flattening your belly. You are in charge of your workout. I'm telling you what to do and how to do it, but you have to want it for yourself. I want you to get rid of any negative thoughts for at least the next 32 days and replace them with positive, affirming thoughts.

You can write these thoughts in a notepad or start a document on your computer. You can also make a copy of the journal in this book. And it doesn't matter if you're not a great writer. It doesn't even matter whether or not you practice proper grammar or spelling. Nobody else is going to read this. Write down anything you want, sentences or notes or whatever, for at least 5 minutes every day. And by working on this every day, you can make sure that all of your future thoughts will be positive, too!

4-Day Jump Start

As you begin the 4-Day Jump Start, observe how you feel about working out. Think about the different yoga poses. Did you have any favorites that stretched muscles you didn't even know you needed? How did you enjoy breaking up your day with Heart Walks? Did you take a break from your TV set to do a lap or two around the block? Use the spaces below to focus on your workouts—and the accomplishments you've achieved—during this time.

DAY 1

Write about how it felt to work out today. Were you out of breath? Did you have to overcome any negative thoughts? Do you now have that exercise high?

_____

_____

_____

_____

_____

_____

_____

_____

_____

DAY 2

Go through your daily schedule and figure out when you can make time for your workouts. Is it easier for you to fit in your workouts first thing in the morning before work? Maybe you can use your lunch hour. Or maybe you have some free time before dinner. Think about what works best for you and write down your new routine.

_____

_____

_____

_____

DAY 3

List four of your health and fitness goals. Be specific. Why did you pick up this book, and what results do you want to see by Day 28?

DAY 4

Today is the last day of your Jump Start—are you ready to bump up your workout tomorrow? If not, how can you prepare yourself?

Your Jump-Start Success

You have completed the first part of your Flat Belly Yoga! workout plan—the 4-Day Jump Start. Take a few minutes to weigh and measure yourself. You are going to be headed into the main phase of your workout program, so I want you to get a gauge on where you are. Did you lose any weight or inches? Don't worry if you didn't. We are about to increase the intensity in your workouts, both in your Heart Walks and by adding weights to your yoga routine (the Core+ workouts), so you're sure to see some changes in the next few weeks.

Before beginning the 4-Week Workout, take a moment to complete a self-evaluation. What was the hardest part of the 4-Day Jump Start? Was it easier than you thought it would be? What time of the day was the easiest for you to work out? What got in your way? Answer these questions below, and use this knowledge to help you succeed during the next 4 weeks.

The 4-Week Workout

Focusing on your goals and the positive results you're seeing day-to-day is a big motivation to stay on track during the 4-Week Workout. So for each day during the next 4 weeks, I've provided you with a Core Confidence, to help you focus each day's entry on the positive impacts of the plan. It's important to blast away those negative thoughts and replace them with positive, affirming words that will help give you the confidence you need to successfully tackle your workouts every day. And each Core Confidence builds upon the ones before it, so be sure to periodically look back and read what you've written in previous entries to help you really track your progress.

DAY 1

CORE CONFIDENCE: What motivated you to pick up *Flat Belly Yoga!*? What results do you want to see by the end of the program? Maybe you want to drop a dress size, have more energy, or look better with your clothes off. Whatever your goal, keep a note of it here to review on days you want to trade in your weights for an extra 10 minutes of sleep.

DAY 2

CORE CONFIDENCE: It can be hard to maintain a workout routine when life gets in the way. What's stopped you in the past? List three things that will help you succeed in putting yourself, and your health, first. Then write down a motivational phrase you can repeat to yourself when you're tempted to give something else priority over your workouts.

_____

_____

_____

_____

_____

_____

_____

_____

_____

_____

DAY 3

CORE CONFIDENCE: Think about how you feel before and after your workout. Do you feel energized in the hours following your Core+ routine? Is it helping you get rid of some of your stress? Write about all the positive feelings that result from your Heart Walks and Core+ routines.

_____

_____

_____

_____

_____

_____

_____

_____

_____

_____

DAY 4

CORE CONFIDENCE: It's important to keep your workouts interesting. On the left-hand side of the page, list three things you enjoy the most about your workout. Next to this, list three ways you can make it even more enjoyable, like adding music or finding a workout buddy. What are you going to do to make that happen? (Examples: making a playlist, calling a friend to work out with you.)

DAY 5

CORE CONFIDENCE: Even if you're not on the Flat Belly Diet! while following the workout plan, you may have noticed a difference in your eating habits. You may find that you're making healthier meal choices after completing your daily workouts. Or maybe the workouts have changed your appetite because you're using up more energy now. Are you hungrier after you work out? Are you craving different foods? Write about how your new routine has affected your diet.

DAY 6

CORE CONFIDENCE: Have a "me day." In every decision, make sure you think about yourself first, especially if you are used to putting everybody else's needs before your own. How does that make you feel?

_____

_____

_____

_____

_____

_____

_____

_____

_____

_____

_____

DAY 7

CORE CONFIDENCE: Today is your last day of Week 1! What were the hardest parts? How can you make them easier in Week 2? For example, if it was hard to make time to work out, what can you change about your schedule? How can you break up your workouts to fit them into your day? If you felt a lot of soreness, what can you do to be more aware of your body while you're working out?

_____

_____

_____

_____

_____

_____

_____

_____

_____

_____

DAY 8

CORE CONFIDENCE: List four things you could give up in place of your workout. Do you really need to watch those late-night TV shows you don't even like? Could you do a 15-minute Core+ workout instead of logging onto Facebook?

DAY 9

CORE CONFIDENCE: List three things to help give you the extra pick-me-up during your Heart Walk. For example, you could pretend a friend of yours is a block away and you are trying to catch up to her. Or if you're listening to music, pick a fast song and try to match your steps to the beat.

DAY 10

CORE CONFIDENCE: Think back over the last few days. Have you had more energy? Are you less irritable? Are you sleeping more soundly and waking up rested? Make a note of how these 10 days have impacted your mood and productivity—you may be surprised to discover the additional benefits of your Core+ workouts.

_____

_____

_____

_____

_____

_____

_____

_____

DAY 11

CORE CONFIDENCE: Focus on your mind-belly connection by using your willpower to help get you through tough workouts. If you had a late night and find you're not looking forward to working out, take a few seconds to adjust your attitude. Look back at your Core Confidence from Day 1 and think about your motivation or inspiration. Write about how you're getting closer to your goal—and remind yourself that your workouts are the reason why.

_____

_____

_____

_____

_____

_____

_____

_____

DAY 12

CORE CONFIDENCE: Research shows that making your goals public makes you much more likely to stick with a plan. So find your own "fan club." Tell your friends or co-workers about your goal and let them cheer you on. It will keep you accountable—and more than that, it will make you *feel* accountable.

DAY 13

CORE CONFIDENCE: What's the one outfit you wish you could still wear? A pair of skinny jeans? How about an elegant cocktail dress? Visualize fitting into it and write about how it would make you feel.

DAY 14

CORE CONFIDENCE: You've made it to the end of Week 2. Congratulations! Write down any changes you have noticed in your body. Can you feel the muscles in your belly yet? Are those pants starting to feel a little looser? And don't forget about your strength-building workouts: Are you feeling stronger in any of the poses? Use the space below to chart your progress up to this point.

_____

_____

_____

_____

_____

_____

_____

_____

_____

_____

DAY 15

CORE CONFIDENCE: Take a long look at yourself in the mirror. How has your body changed? What do you see, or not see? Focus on positive thoughts and changes. It's important to reinforce all of your good behavior to keep you on track for the next 2 weeks.

_____

_____

_____

_____

_____

_____

_____

_____

_____

DAY 16

CORE CONFIDENCE: This week, you were introduced to several new poses in the Core+ 20-Minute Workout Routine. Which one was your favorite and why? How can you make the other poses as much fun as this one?

_____

_____

_____

_____

_____

_____

_____

_____

_____

DAY 17

CORE CONFIDENCE: Is there an activity you've always wanted to do but have been afraid to try? Maybe now is the time for you to give it a shot. If you're still apprehensive, think about how your workouts for the last 16 days have helped to prepare you, either physically, mentally, or both. Describe what you can do for the next 11 days to help you reach this goal.

_____

_____

_____

_____

_____

_____

_____

_____

DAY 18

CORE CONFIDENCE: Try to incorporate some new tunes into your workout, whether it's for your Heart Walk or Core+ workout. Research shows that music can improve your workout by giving you more energy. So maybe a new beat is just what you need to keep you jamming along. After your workout, write about whether or not you noticed a difference with your new music.

_____

_____

_____

_____

_____

_____

_____

_____

_____

_____

DAY 19

CORE CONFIDENCE: Write down four of your best attributes. Say them 10 times now, and repeat them anytime negative thoughts appear. Your goal is to shut down your inner critic.

_____

_____

_____

_____

_____

_____

_____

_____

_____

_____

DAY 20

CORE CONFIDENCE: Switch up the timing of your walk today. If you usually go out in the evening, take advantage of your lunch break and soak up some vitamin D in the form of sunshine. Or if you usually get sweaty first thing in the morning, go enjoy the cool of dusk. This simple switch-up can make your Heart Walk more interesting and fun. Did it work?

DAY 21

CORE CONFIDENCE: It's the end of Week 3. Can you believe how far you've come? Write about how it feels to stick with the plan for this long. Are you proud of yourself? You should be! You made goals and you stuck to them. Even if you didn't do everything perfectly, congratulate yourself for having come this far.

DAY 22

CORE CONFIDENCE: You've made it to Week 4! Write down all the compliments you have received, even (especially) the ones you've given yourself. (Example: "Wow, I look great!")

_____

_____

_____

_____

_____

_____

_____

_____

_____

_____

_____

DAY 23

CORE CONFIDENCE: Now it's time to "get naked." I know this can be intimidating, but take off your clothes and describe what you see in the mirror. Focus on the positive. What's getting better? What can you see changing?

_____

_____

_____

_____

_____

_____

_____

_____

_____

_____

_____

_____

DAY 24

CORE CONFIDENCE: Now that you've been working out for 24 days, think about your motives to continue with the program. What are your new goals? How do they compare with the ones you had when you started? You may be surprised to see how much they've changed!

_____

_____

_____

_____

_____

_____

_____

_____

DAY 25

CORE CONFIDENCE: Take a look at your "before picture." Okay, you have three more days until the end of the program. How can you put a little more energy into your workout to make your "after picture" the best it can be? Write down three things you can do, such as pushing yourself to walk a little faster or holding your poses a few seconds longer.

_____

_____

_____

_____

_____

_____

_____

_____

DAY 26

CORE CONFIDENCE: Start writing your success story. Where were you when you decided to pick up this book? How did you feel about yourself? What obstacles did you have to overcome as you started your 4-Day Jump Start? Are they still obstacles? How did working out feel at the start? How is it now? Has it gotten easier and become a part of your routine?

DAY 27

CORE CONFIDENCE: Think back to Day 1 of the 4-Day Jump Start. How has your life changed for the better? Do you feel less stressed now? Do the little things make you less angry? Are you sleeping better? Do you have more energy? List everything you can think of. (The small things count, too!)

DAY 28

CORE CONFIDENCE: Congratulations, you have successfully completed the Flat Belly Yoga! program. I want you to step on the scale and measure yourself. Be proud of your progress. You stuck with it and you did the work. Describe how it feels to complete this program and reach the goal you set for yourself. Make a promise to yourself that you will continue to practice putting yourself (and your health) first.

Journal Tips

When you are writing your journal, practice what we call *free writing*. Don't stop to think about spelling or grammar. Don't stop to think about whether you are "being a good person" or what someone else would say if they saw this. No one will—in fact, a helpful promise you can make is to agree that no one is going to see this but you. Now you have no pressure to write in a certain way or the "right way." Give yourself this gift: Just be honest with yourself.

A FLAT BELLY YOGA
SUCCESS STORY

Kelly Boyer

Age: 48

Pounds lost:

6

in 32 days

All-over inches lost:

8.5

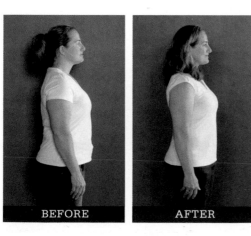

BEFORE · AFTER

" I was ready for a change," states Kelly Boyer, an amateur body builder for the last 6 years. Having been active for most of her life, Kelly's heavy lifting began taking a toll on her body. "My body has sustained a lot of injuries—particularly my shoulders, which are held together with pins and screws. I was at a loss as to how to address the problem while maintaining a reasonable degree of muscular conditioning," she explains.

So when Kelly found out about the Flat Belly Yoga! Workout, she followed her instincts that this was exactly what she'd been looking for and jumped at the chance to begin the workout. "I literally became aware of the program and agreed to participate in it within a 2.5-hour time frame," she exclaims. "I wanted to find a new exercise regimen that I could age into that would not be hard on my body."

The 48-year-old body builder says that while the routine of the program was easy for her to follow, mastering the yoga poses was a little difficult. But she quickly learned how adaptable yoga can be. Due to her injuries, Kelly used some alternate poses to avoid additional stress to those specific areas (see the *Mat Matters* tips throughout the book for several alternate poses).

But even though Kelly's injuries prevented her from completing the full poses, she didn't let that affect her motivation. To make sure she stayed on track throughout the 32-day program, she wrote diligently in her journal. "Journaling helped me stay focused by reminding me why I started the program, which was the lifestyle change that I knew

I wanted," she says. "I wanted to be ache-free, flexible, toned, less stressed. I wrote about the changes I saw in my body, attitude, emotions, etc., in my journal. And it was there that I realized I was succeeding."

Each day, Kelly set a goal for herself and wrote it in her journal. She would then follow up with probing questions. "I would ask myself if I was doing everything I could to be successful," she describes. "Was I pushing myself? Was I taking it too easy? I wrote about struggling with certain poses and getting into them in a timely manner." And when she reached her goals, Kelly knew the importance of celebrating those milestones by writing how proud she was of herself.

And she was grateful to have those handwritten notes when she reached a roadblock during her journey. "I reached a point where I was incredibly tired," she says. "That was the first point where I read what I had written in my journal from the beginning. I looked for—and found—the nuggets of success that helped me stay focused and move forward. I realized that I was only tired because I was succeeding—changing your life is not an easy task."

Kelly says that while the future looks bright, she still has some work to do. "I am starting a second round of the program that I am calling Boyer Boot Camp," she smiles. "I plan to journal the entire time and will ask my friends to submit questions for me to respond to. So, I guess journaling and exercise now go hand-in-hand for me. I'm very much looking forward to it. It's a very good life I have been given."

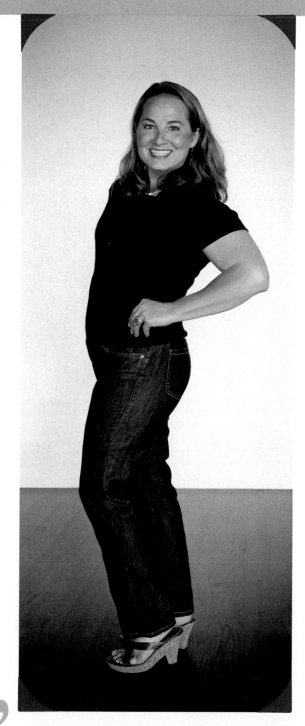

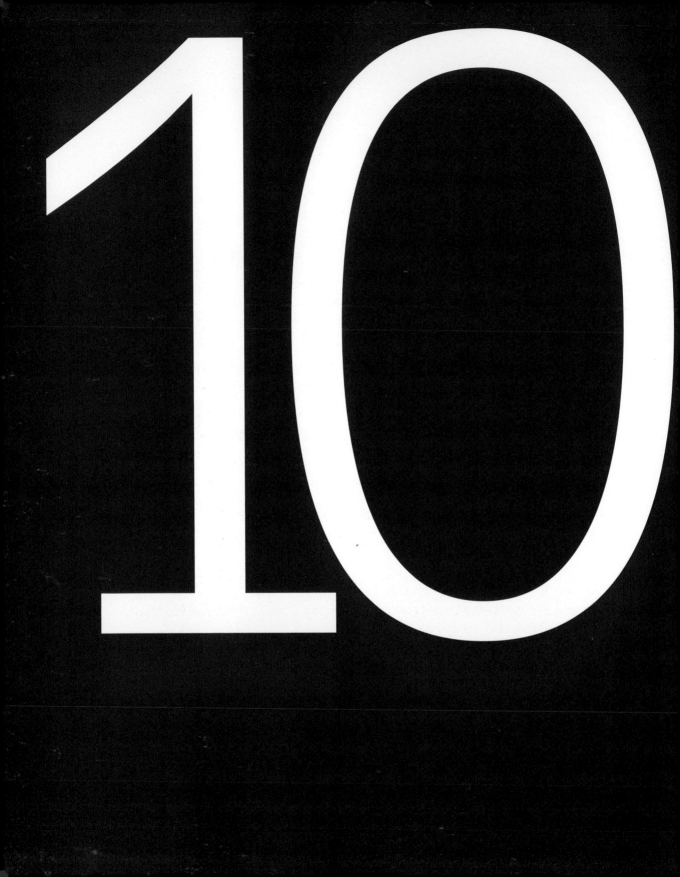

THE FLAT BELLY DIET! CHEAT SHEET

The Flat Belly Yoga! Workout can give you the midsection of your dreams. But combining it with the Flat Belly Diet! will give you even better results. In fact, this workout program was actually designed to work alongside the diet plan, and is even structured the same way as the diet, with a 4-Day Jump Start followed by a 4-Week Plan.

If you haven't read *Prevention* magazine's *New York Times* bestselling book, *Flat Belly Diet!*, I would suggest picking it up, or go to www.flatbellydiet.com for more information. I'm going to give you a condensed version ("cheat sheet") with at-a-glance information such as:

- An introduction to the new science of conquering belly fat with MUFAs
- An overview of the rules and guidelines of the diet
- A look at the delicious and familiar foods at the center of the diet
- A breakdown of the 4-Day Anti-Bloat Jump Start and the 4-Week Plan
- Sample recipes and techniques that will help you change your grocery shopping and eating habits

Diet and Exercise: A Winning Combination

There's no question that you will see dramatic improvements in your health and strength by doing the workout alone. By following the Flat Belly Yoga! program, you'll reduce dangerous belly fat, strengthen your core, and be healthier and more energetic.

But why not combine your new exercise program with the perfect complement—a diet that was designed to reach the same objectives? A diet that will help you reach your flat belly goal faster? A diet that will strengthen your ability to maintain the new, healthier you?

As we discussed in the Introduction, scientific studies have proved that when it comes to losing weight and keeping it off, diet or exercise alone are no match for the combination of the two. If you prefer, you can flatten your belly simply by following the Flat Belly Yoga! program on its own. But by using the two together, you can get the best possible result: You'll stack benefit on top of benefit—and double your sense of accomplishment.

MUFAs Matter

The relationship between the fat in our diet and the fat on our bellies isn't as simple as it sounds. We want to eliminate dangerous belly fat, but nutritionally

Getting the Most Out of MUFAs

Monounsaturated fatty acids (MUFAs) are the core building blocks of the Flat Belly Diet! But what exactly are MUFAs?

We hear a lot about saturated and unsaturated fats. And if you think about the name, it's easy to remember why unsaturated fats are healthier.

Fats are chains of carbon and hydrogen atoms. In a molecule of **saturated fat,** every carbon atom is connected to a hydrogen atom. At room temperature, the fat is waxy or solid. And inside of your body, the fat is sticky and tough. Think of a towel that's saturated with water on a hot, humid day—that towel's not going to dry out for a long time.

An **unsaturated fat** isn't as tightly constructed as a saturated fat. It's more flexible and less likely to cause blockages as it moves throughout your body, which makes them the healthier option.

MUFAs, a type of unsaturated fat, move through your bloodstream with ease and grace. Not only do they have none of the clogging effects of saturated fats, they actually help protect your arteries from harmful buildup.

At the same time, the carbs and proteins that you eat trigger the release of insulin. Because belly fat leads to higher levels of cortisol and adrenaline that work against insulin, your insulin levels rise to keep up with those stress hormones. And when insulin rises, fat sticks to your middle.

But unlike saturated fat, MUFAs tend to lower insulin levels—turning the vicious cycle of increased belly fat into a healthy nutritional balance that helps you slim down.

Rich in plant-based antioxidants, fiber, and other healthy nutrients, the components of this diet don't only fight belly fat. They also ward off heart disease, type 2 diabetes, high blood pressure, and cancer. Each individual component has additional benefits, too. The antioxidants and resveratrol in nuts and dark chocolate, the oleocanthal in olive oil, and the beta-sitosterol in avocados all help your body stay healthy in different ways.

speaking, fats remain a critical component of a healthy diet. The trick is learning which fats we can count on for nourishment and which to avoid.

The Flat Belly Diet! is built around the healthy oils found in many plant foods, known as MUFAs, or *monounsaturated fatty acids*. (For more of the science behind MUFAs, see "Getting the Most Out of MUFAs" on page 207.)

There are five basic categories of MUFAs, and guess what? *They're delicious!* If you've been turned off of dieting because you believe that food is one of the pleasures of life, you will feel at home on the Flat Belly Diet! because you don't have to sacrifice good-tasting foods. These five MUFAs are your allies on the path to a flat belly:

- Oils
- Nuts and seeds
- Avocados
- Olives
- Dark chocolate

That's a range of rich, sensuous tastes that not too many people associate with the word *diet*. They come from the centuries-old Mediterranean diet— a healthy, traditional lifestyle that prevents disease and leads to optimal health.

So let's see how the diet incorporates those foods, and all of their health benefits, into a pleasurable, *achievable* nutritional program.

The Rules

These three simple rules structure the Flat Belly Diet!:

Rule 1: STICK TO 400 CALORIES PER MEAL.

The meals and snacks in this diet, based around MUFAs and other wholesome foods, all total around 400 calories per meal. It's all right to use this number as a daily average rather than a strict limit for every meal—just make sure your total caloric intake is around 1,600 calories per day. If you have a big lunch, it's okay to have a slightly smaller snack, or vice versa.

Some diets restrict caloric intake even further. That's not healthy, and it's not sustainable. Sixteen-hundred calories is a healthy target for daily eating, one that you can hit well after the 32 days of the Flat Belly Diet!.

Rule 2: NEVER GO MORE THAN 4 HOURS WITHOUT EATING.

Would you rather feel hungry and tired—or fueled and energized? Eating at regular hours with not too much time in between will keep your metabolism in a healthy gear. Instead of being assailed by diet-destroying cravings, you will feel revved up, and you'll burn calories throughout the day.

Rule 3: INCLUDE A MUFA AT EVERY MEAL.

You already know the benefits of MUFAs. I'll give you a few starter ideas for meal planning around MUFAs, but to really see the full range of recipes available to you, I recommend getting your hands on a copy of the *Flat Belly Diet! Cookbook*. (The *Flat Belly Diet! Pocket Guide* and the original *Flat Belly Diet!* also have pages of recipes, shopping lists, and daily meal plans built around MUFAs and other tasty, nutritious foods.)

The Guidelines

In addition to the three rules above, these four guidelines will help you create healthy meals and accomplish your Flat Belly! goals.

Guideline 1: CONSUME NO MORE THAN 4 GRAMS OF SATURATED FAT PER MEAL.

Saturated fat (remember that wet towel?) causes all sorts of problems. It raises your LDL, the "bad" cholesterol, and it increases your risk of cardiovascular disease and stroke. You'll find a lot of saturated fats in animal products like meat and dairy, as well as in tropical oils like coconut oil, palm oil, or palm kernel oil. Cocoa butter is also a source of high amounts of saturated fats.

You can't eliminate saturated fats from your diet entirely—you'll consume small amounts in many different plant foods, including MUFA-rich foods such as olive oil and nuts. But it's easy to find healthy alternatives. Avoid butter in favor of substituting healthier fats like olive oil or canola oil. The recipes in the *Flat Belly Diet!* will help you limit your saturated fat intake to around 3 grams per meal.

Guideline 2: BAN TRANS FATS.

Not only do trans fats increase your LDL, they also lower your HDL, the "good" cholesterol that keeps your blood vessels clear. You'll find trans fats in packaged products that are manufactured to sit on store shelves. They're made by adding hydrogen to liquid oils to make them solid, which extends shelf life. Food regulations allow manufacturers to say a product has zero trans fats even when it contains up to half a gram per serving. So scan the ingredients for the words *hydrogenated, partially hydrogenated,* or *shortening* to make sure you're not innocently ingesting trans fats in small amounts, which can add up.

Guideline 3: AVOID ARTIFICIAL SWEETENERS, FLAVORINGS, AND PRESERVATIVES.

Reading the ingredients in your food choices shouldn't make you feel like you're doing graduate-level chemistry research. Choose whole foods whenever you can, and look for ingredients you can recognize and pronounce. Here are a couple of bad pennies that turn up time and time again:

- Aspartame is an artificial sweetener often found in diet sodas, sugar-free yogurts and puddings, chewable vitamins, gum, and high-fiber cereal. Although the Food and Drug Administration approved it for use more than 30 years ago, its safety is questionable, as it's been linked to headaches, dizziness, and mood changes.

- Artificial food colorings have been linked to hyperactivity in children.

- Nitrates, used to add flavor to meats, have been linked to cancer.

Guideline 4: LIMIT SODIUM TO LESS THAN 2,300 MILLIGRAMS A DAY.

Keeping your sodium under 2,300 milligrams a day (575 milligrams per meal) will speed you toward two goals: having a flatter belly and being healthier. As you reduce sodium, you'll stop retaining water and begin losing pounds and unsightly puffiness. Another reason to cut salt from your diet is that high sodium also contributes to heart and kidney disease. It also raises your chances of having a stroke.

The Secret to Your Success

Three rules. Four guidelines. That's not too much to keep in mind!

You'll find that the Flat Belly Diet! has a crucial element in common with the Flat Belly Yoga! program: They both have simple instructions. The diet's prescriptions are backed by scientific research. And its plans make logical sense, so it's easy to follow and maintain the eating plan.

Here are four reasons are why I believe that the Flat Belly Diet!, like the Flat Belly Yoga! program, can become a permanent part of your recipe for health:

- *It's built on healthy foods.* This isn't about a list of branded, prepackaged items. And it isn't about trendy supplements, shakes, or juices. It's about eating natural foods that have kept people healthy for centuries.

- *It's not "low calorie."* The average woman over 40 needs 1,600 calories a day to maintain a healthy weight, which is why that's the basis for the Flat Belly Diet! (You can use the online calculator at www.flatbellydiet.com to tailor the diet to your age, gender, and activity level.) This is not a diet that only allows you to have morsels spaced out far apart, which will make you feel sad and hungry. Meals are designed to be filling and frequent to keep you energized and alert.

- *It tastes good.* The building blocks of the Flat Belly Diet! are avocados, oils, nuts and seeds, olives, and dark chocolate. If you saw that selection on a menu, the first word to come to mind wouldn't be *diet*.

- *It's easy.* Breakfast, lunch, dinner, and snacks are each designed at 400 calories, so it's easy to switch foods around for variety. With the Flat Belly Diet! books, you'll get individual calorie breakdowns that will help you build endless menus by mixing and matching your favorite foods.

Finally, one other element makes the Flat Belly Diet! a recipe for success: *Almost nothing is forbidden.* You'll learn how to build meals around MUFAs and how to pair them with carbohydrates and proteins ranging from whole grains and fruits to lean meats. But the fact is, you don't have to give up your favorite foods to start the Flat Belly Diet!. You just have to eat them according to the three rules and four guidelines we discussed earlier.

So are you ready to turbocharge your Flat Belly Yoga! Workout with a diet that will compound your chances of success? Let's get started!

The Jump Start: 4 Days to Beat Bloat

If you are combining the Flat Belly Diet! with the Flat Belly Yoga! Workout, make sure to do the two Jump Starts together. Don't go straight into the 4-Week Meal Plan. The first 4 days of the diet are a transitional period during which you will be eating smaller meals and cleansing your system. So don't overlap the 4-Day Anti-Bloat Jump Start of the diet with the 4-Week Workout in *Flat Belly Yoga!* because you won't be eating enough calories to give you the energy you'll need for the workouts.

Part of what makes these two programs so strong together is that they both contain a 4-Day Jump Start followed by a 4-Week Plan. They'll work best when those corresponding components are aligned as two phases of one energizing challenge because the workouts were designed with the diet in mind. More importantly, by lining up the two programs correctly, you'll feel your best and get the most out of it!

WHY AM I BLOATED?

Bloating isn't just a result of how you eat—it's also reflective of how you live. Consider how you can reduce these bloat-inducing factors as you embark upon the Jump Start.

Stress. It causes certain hormones to fluctuate. They raise your blood pressure, sending blood out into your arms and legs. As blood leaves your core, your digestive system slows to a crawl. Now it's going to take longer to digest that last meal, and the longer it sits in your intestines, the more you bloat. I'm sure you have experienced this—I know I have.

Lack of fluid. It sounds like the reverse might be true, but you need to drink fluids to prevent your body from retaining water. Drink at least 8 glasses of water every day, and supplement your liquid intake with water-rich fruits and vegetables like celery and watermelon.

Lack of sleep. When you deprive yourself of sleep, you throw your body out of whack in many ways—one of which is digestion. Get a full night's rest so you can count on your GI tract to do its work properly.

Air travel. As cabin pressure drops, the air and gases inside your body—specifically, inside your digestive tract—expand. Your body, confused by rapid environmental changes, retains water. You can't always avoid air travel, but you can make sure to drink extra water. Plus, you can stretch your legs and take short walks up and down the aisle during the flight.

How to Jump-Start Your Diet

By keeping the following five principles in mind as you go through your 4-Day Anti-Bloat Jump Start, you will emerge on the other side refreshed, energized, and ready to continue with the 4-Week Plans.

Jump Start Principle 1: FOLLOW THE 4-DAY MEAL PLAN.

I've included all four days of the Jump Start menu from *Flat Belly Diet!* for your convenience. (See the Jump Start Menu Day 1 on page 216.)

The foods you'll be eating are not the same foods that make up the 4-Week Meal Plan in the *Flat Belly Diet!* As you can see on the "Banned!" list (see "Banned! The No-Go List for Your Jump Start" on page 215), lots of nutritious, tasty foods can contribute to bloating. But once you incorporate them into a balanced, MUFA-rich diet, you'll be able to control bloat. In fact, some of these foods are main ingredients in the meals you'll be eating over the following 28 days. But for these 4 days, I want you to focus on reducing your belly bloat.

There are some restrictions, but the Flat Belly Diet! has a menu plan that contains the nutrition you need to reduce bloat and tastes good enough to help you reduce the salt and artificial flavorings you're putting into your body.

Jump Start Principle 2: EAT FOUR 300-CALORIE MEALS A DAY.

There are two important elements to this. The first is getting you on a schedule of eating four meals a day, including your afternoon snack. The second is making sure there's less food overall in your system, giving it a chance to clear out bloat without getting backed up. The series of four 1,200-calorie days is the main reason I recommend combining both programs' 4-Day Jump Starts. Take it easy on yourself now. You'll get a chance to push yourself—and enjoy the results from doing so—later.

Jump Start Principle 3: DRINK ONE FULL BATCH OF SASSY WATER EACH DAY.

Sassy Water is the signature beverage recipe from the Flat Belly Diet!, invented by coauthor Cynthia Sass. It's a perky treat that helps soothe your GI tract with the bright taste of ginger.

The night before each day of the Jump Start, you're going to make a full recipe and drink it over the course of the next day. Its unique flavor will remind you that the 4 days of your Jump Start are a doorway to changing your health, your body, and your life.

Sassy Water Recipe

2 liters water (about 8½ cups)
1 teaspoon freshly grated ginger
1 medium cucumber, peeled and thinly sliced
1 medium lemon, thinly sliced
12 small spearmint leaves

Combine all ingredients in a large pitcher and let flavors blend overnight. Drink the entire pitcher by the end of each day.

Jump Start Principle 4: EAT SLOWLY.

Slow down! When you eat too quickly, you swallow huge gulps of air with your meal. There's no calorie cost to a mouthful of air, but it gets trapped in your digestive system. And slowing down to eat will decrease the stress that leads to bloating, too.

Jump Start Principle 5: AVOID THESE FOODS.

The foods on the "Banned!" list have the potential to increase bloat. As we discussed earlier these aren't bad foods. You're just going to take a little break from them in order to focus on belly bloat and get ready for your 4-Week Meal Plan.

Banned! The No-Go List for Your Jump Start

The following foods are off-limits during the 4-Day Anti-Bloat Jump Start:

- Alcohol, coffee, tea, hot cocoa, and acidic fruit juices
- Bulky raw foods
- Carbonated beverages
- Chewing gum
- Excess carbs
- Fatty foods
- Fried foods
- Gassy foods, including broccoli, Brussels sprouts, cabbage, cauliflower, citrus fruits, legumes, onions, and peppers
- Salt, including salt from the saltshaker, salt-based seasonings, and highly processed foods
- Spicy foods, including foods seasoned with barbecue sauce, black pepper, chili peppers, chili powder, cloves, garlic, horseradish, hot sauce, ketchup, mustard, nutmeg, onions, tomato sauce, or vinegar
- Sugar alcohols, such as xylitol and maltitol, which are often found in low-calorie, low-carb, or sugar-free products such as candy, chewing gum, ice cream, and jam

BREAKFAST

1 cup unsweetened cornflakes

1 cup fat-free milk

$\frac{1}{4}$ cup roasted or raw unsalted sunflower seeds

4 ounces ($\frac{1}{2}$ cup) unsweetened applesauce

Glass of Sassy Water

LUNCH

4 ounces deli turkey

1 pint fresh grape tomatoes

1 low-fat string cheese

Glass of Sassy Water

SNACK

Blueberry Smoothie: Blend 1 cup fat-free milk and 1 cup frozen unsweetened blueberries in a blender for 1 minute. Transfer to a glass and stir in 1 tablespoon cold-pressed organic flaxseed oil or serve with 2 tablespoons sunflower seeds, without the shell.

DINNER

4 ounces grilled tilapia, drizzled with 1 teaspoon olive oil

1 cup steamed green beans

$\frac{1}{2}$ cup cooked brown rice

Glass of Sassy Water

BREAKFAST

1 packet instant Cream of Wheat

1 cup fat-free milk

¼ cup roasted or raw unsalted sunflower seeds

2 tablespoons unsweetened raisins

Glass of Sassy Water

LUNCH

3 ounces chunk light tuna in water, drained

1 cup steamed baby carrots

1 low-fat string cheese

Glass of Sassy Water

SNACK

Pineapple Smoothie: Blend 1 cup fat-free milk,
4 ounces canned pineapple tidbits in juice, and a handful
of ice in a blender for 1 minute. Transfer to a glass and stir
in 1 tablespoon cold-pressed organic flaxseed oil or serve
with 2 tablespoons sunflower seeds, without the shell.

DINNER

3 ounces grilled chicken breast, drizzled with
1 teaspoon olive oil

1 cup cremini mushrooms, sauteed in cooking spray,
if desired

½ cup cooked brown rice

Glass of Sassy Water

BREAKFAST

1 cup unsweetened cornflakes

1 cup fat-free milk

¼ cup roasted or raw unsalted sunflower seeds

2 tablespoons unsweetened raisins

Glass of Sassy Water

LUNCH

4 ounces deli turkey

1 cup steamed baby carrots

1 low-fat string cheese

Glass of Sassy Water

SNACK

Blueberry Smoothie: Blend 1 cup fat-free milk and 1 cup frozen unsweetened blueberries in a blender for 1 minute. Transfer to a glass and stir in 1 tablespoon cold-pressed organic flaxseed oil or serve with 2 tablespoons sunflower seeds, without the shell.

DINNER

4 ounces grilled tilapia, drizzled with 1 teaspoon olive oil

1 cup cremini mushrooms, sauteed in cooking spray, if desired

½ cup cooked brown rice

Glass of Sassy Water

BREAKFAST

1 packet instant Cream of Wheat

1 cup fat-free milk

¼ cup roasted or raw unsalted sunflower seeds

4 ounces (½ cup) unsweetened applesauce

Glass of Sassy Water

LUNCH

3 ounces chunk light tuna in water, drained

1 pint fresh grape tomatoes

1 low-fat string cheese

Glass of Sassy Water

SNACK

Pineapple Smoothie: Blend 1 cup fat-free milk, 4 ounces canned pineapple tidbits in juice, and a handful of ice in a blender for 1 minute. Transfer to a glass and stir in 1 tablespoon cold-pressed organic flaxseed oil or serve with 2 tablespoons sunflower seeds, without the shell.

DINNER

3 ounces grilled chicken breast, drizzled with 1 teaspoon olive oil

1 cup steamed green beans

½ cup cooked brown rice

Glass of Sassy Water

Jump Start Menu Day 4

THE 4-WEEK MEAL PLAN

Just like with the 4-Week Flat Belly Yoga! Workout, the Flat Belly Diet! is something you can make a part of your daily life to ensure years of loving the way you look and feel. But it's the change you'll feel after the first 28 days that will flip a switch—it will convince you that you can beat belly fat with a daily routine that's achievable, fun, and delicious.

MAKING MUFAS INTO MEALS

After you've completed the 4 days of the Anti-Bloat Jump Start, you're going to feel different. You're going to feel significantly less bloated, clearer-headed, and less sluggish. And if you've accomplished the 4-day Flat Belly Yoga! Jump Start at the same time, you'll probably feel pretty unstoppable.

But after 4 days, you'll also be ready for a change. Now it's time to ease back into a wider, less restricted range of healthy eating. You can tear up the banned foods list. Many people find they aren't as interested in fried food or chewing gum after they've completed the no-nonsense Jump Start.

But if something on the banned list means a lot to you, rest assured that in the right amounts, you can incorporate it into the flexible, scientifically sound 4-Week Meal Plan—as well as into your regular diet afterwards. (And remember—plenty of those banned foods are very healthy. You only had to cut them out for an anti-bloat boost.)

The *Flat Belly Diet!* contains pages of delicious menus. But it contains something even more important: The tools to shape healthy meals that you can share with friends and family long after you've completed your 4-Week Meal Plan. And it shows you how to master creating meals out of simple building blocks.

To summarize, you'll start with a MUFA. You'll add lean protein, vegetables, low-fat dairy, and starches. Every time you do it, you'll wind up with a new variation on an old theme—the legendary Mediterranean diet. And after you've done it for 28 days, you'll have broadened your health food horizons, so your options will be truly limitless.

GET TO KNOW YOUR MUFAS

Oils, nuts and seeds, avocados, olives, and dark chocolate. These are five delicious kinds of MUFAs that you can use as building blocks to make a terrific assortment of tasty meals. Let's discuss each one in a little more detail to give you a picture about the kinds of meals and snacks available to you. The closer you look at each MUFA-rich element, the more options you're going to find.

You can count on *Flat Belly Diet!*, *Flat Belly Diet! Pocket Guide*, and *Flat Belly Diet! Cookbook* to provide endless menus and recipes for you to enjoy. But to make it easy for you, I am going to give you an idea of some of the delicious possibilities awaiting you.

NO ALL-MUFA MEALS!

MUFAs are calorie-dense foods. So keep in mind that they're only building blocks for meals—not meals in themselves. MUFAs are helpful, healthy foods, but balance them with lean protein and healthy carbs, as shown here.

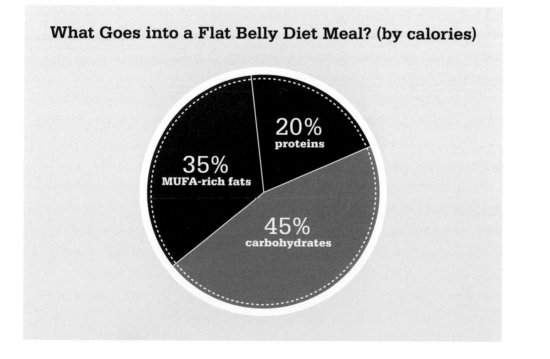

What Goes into a Flat Belly Diet Meal? (by calories)

20% proteins

35% MUFA-rich fats

45% carbohydrates

MUFA 1: Oils

Oils have a lot of negative associations, but a tasty serving of plant-based oil is a great way to introduce an element of MUFA goodness into an ordinary meal.

When shopping for oils, look for expeller-pressed or cold-pressed oils. Oils can become rancid, so purchase them in amounts small enough to use in a couple of months. And store them in a cool, dark place, such as your pantry or refrigerator. Refrigerated oils may thicken as they cool, but this doesn't hurt them at all. They'll return to liquid form after they've been at room temperature for a little while.

There are many ways to include MUFA-rich oils in your diet. Drizzle **extra virgin olive oil** on salads, vegetables, meats, and fish just as you would use a flavoring on a finished meal. Or use a less-expensive olive oil to sauté food on your stovetop with moderate heat.

Canola oil should be used for baking or in recipes that call for stovetop heating with moderately high heat.

Refined peanut oil is good for higher-temperature cooking.

Sesame oil has strong flavor and adds an intense taste to marinades, dipping sauces, dressings, and especially stir-fries.

High-oleic safflower and sunflower oils are great for cold salads—they don't congeal as quickly as other oils. And *high-oleic* means they've been especially formulated to be higher in MUFAs!

Walnut oil is an expensive, flavorful oil good for use in specialty dishes.

Flaxseed oil is delicious when it's cold. You can add it to salads or smoothies or swirl it into a cold soup. Heating it destroys its nutritional properties, so don't use it when cooking meals.

MUFA 2: Nuts and Seeds

Shop for whole nuts to ensure freshness and save money. With their shells intact, nuts will retain their nutritional content. They're hardy, too—you can keep whole nuts in a cool, dark place for 2 to 3 months. Shelled nuts are delicious and nutritious, but buy them unsalted, raw, or roasted without oil. You can keep them in the refrigerator for up to 4 months.

Nuts are a great on-the-go snack food. A standard serving size for nuts is

2 tablespoons. You can measure that quantity into plastic bags to take with you, or carry a larger package and a tablespoon. And different nuts may go well with different dishes. Consider throwing sliced **almonds** into a salad, chopping **Brazil nuts** into a pilaf or grain-based salad, using **cashews** in a curry, mixing **hazelnuts** into your granola, or serving **macadamia nuts** with tropical fruits or even mild fish dishes. Also, **pecans** aren't just for dessert—try them with roasted squash or in pancakes. **Pine nuts** share MUFA duty in pesto, which mixes them with olive oil in a zesty mixture that can be used as a spread or a sauce. Try pairing **pistachios** with chicken or other savory dishes, and keep **walnuts** as a staple—they last two to three times as long as other nuts and are versatile ingredients. You can puree them into a dip or crumble them over a salad.

Nuts are also delicious toasted—a cooking method that requires no additional oil. A toaster oven at 250 degrees Fahrenheit or a pan on low heat will toast nuts in under 4 minutes. As soon as they brown, remove them from the heat—there's no rescuing burned nuts, which immediately turn bitter to the taste.

Two special **legumes** can bring the MUFAs to your table. **Peanuts** can be purchased raw, dry roasted, or boiled (whole or shelled) and store as easily and as long as tree nuts. Peanuts make an easy snack and can be chopped and sprinkled over stir-fries and salads. Of course, peanut butter is a classic sandwich spread and a healthy snack component. (Don't forget about other nut butters, like almond and cashew. They're available in healthful recipes that add very few ingredients—often just a little salt and oil). **Edamame** (green soybeans) are a classic appetizer in Japanese cuisine. They can be purchased fresh at farmers' markets and found in the frozen aisles of large supermarkets. And 1 cup of shelled edamame is a single MUFA serving.

Seeds are a more versatile MUFA. Buy them in bulk at natural foods stores—they will keep in airtight containers for a couple of months. You've probably snacked on roasted pumpkin seeds, but have you ever made your own tahini—a rich Middle Eastern sauce that flavors hummus—from sesame seeds? (It's also available in the ethnic food aisles of most supermarkets.) You can sprinkle seeds over salads, bake them into muffins, or grind them up and fold them into burger mixes or use them as a base in sauces and dips.

MUFA 3: Avocados

The creamy, green flesh of the avocado seems so decadent that it can be surprising how healthy it is for you. Not only is it packed with MUFAs, it's also rich in cancer-fighting carotenoids.

Buy unripe avocados—look for firm fruits that yield very little to a squeeze—and allow them to ripen at room temperature over a day or two. (You can put them in a brown paper bag to speed up this process.) A ripe avocado can be used as a spread on sandwiches and burgers. On the firm side, it stands up as a salad ingredient or as a side dish with a splash of fresh lime. And definitely experiment with **guacamole,** a combination of mashed avocados, chopped onions, jalapeño peppers, cilantro, and lime juice.

MUFA 4: Olives

This classic Mediterranean snack packs a mean MUFA punch. It also contains antioxidant vitamin E, which has many skin-related health benefits. Buy unpasteurized fresh, whole olives rather than pasteurized jarred or canned pitted olives, and keep them in the refrigerator. Snack on them whole or incorporate them into salads or sauces for chicken. Learn how to make **tapenade,** a mix of chopped olives, olive oil, and seasonings that can be used as a spread or a sauce. (Some tapenades replace olives with artichokes or eggplant, which means that however tasty they may be, they don't count as MUFAs. Don't be fooled!)

MUFA 5: Dark Chocolate

You were wondering about this one, weren't you? What kind of a diet lists dark chocolate as not only a permissible treat, but a major building block? The fact is, dark chocolate, with at least **60 percent cacao,** is a perfectly healthy, MUFA-rich food. Store it in a cool, dark place (but not in the refrigerator) and it can last for up to a year. Eat it on its own, swirl it into oatmeal, shave it over fruit, or mix it into pancake, waffle, or muffin batters.

MEALS FROM THE MUFA UP

The recipes you'll find in *Flat Belly Diet!* will help you generate dozens of delicious meals to help you get rid of belly fat. Before you look at a sample breakfast, lunch, snack, and dinner from the 4-Week Meal Plan, take a minute to understand how other ingredients—proteins, vegetables, and carbohydrates—combine with MUFAs to make up your meals.

Lean Protein

Meats are one of the most likely foods where you'll encounter *saturated fats*—and as you remember from your guidelines, you're going to want to avoid those. By picking *lean* proteins, you'll reduce your saturated fat intake and be able to follow the guideline of 3 to 4 grams of saturated fat per meal.

- **Beef, poultry, and pork** are packed with high-quality protein. Make sure to shop for lean cuts of meat, skinless and boneless poultry, and pork loins and hams. Look for 90-percent or higher "lean" ground beef and low-fat ground turkey breast.

- When using **vegetarian substitutes,** check labels to ensure that you're getting no more than 2 grams of saturated fat and 480 milligrams of sodium per serving.

- **Organic meats** tend to be lower in sodium and fat and have other health and environmental benefits.

- **Fish** are full of heart-healthy omega-3 fats, especially the fatty dark fish such as salmon, tuna, and bluefish. Light-colored fish are lower in fat, as are many shellfish, and all provide high-quality protein. Wild-caught fish will have fewer contaminants than farmed fish. When buying canned fish, make sure it is low in sodium and packed in water instead of oil.

- **Egg whites** are naturally free of fat and cholesterol.

- Low-fat or fat-free **dairy products** provide important vitamins and minerals that will help prevent osteoporosis. Just about any dairy product should be available in a low-fat or fat-free version. And milk, yogurt, and cheese are often exactly what a MUFA-rich meal needs for a bit of extra pizzazz. Calcium-fortified **soy** is often a healthy dairy alternative for lactose intolerant or vegan dieters.

Fruits and Vegetables

For delicious tastes and healthy fiber, nothing can replace the role of fruits and vegetables in the Flat Belly Diet!.

Here's just one example of the tasty daily menus you can enjoy during the Flat Belly Diet! 4-Week Meal Plan. MUFAs are in boldface. Calories are in parentheses.

Pick up a copy of *Flat Belly Diet!* or *Flat Belly Diet! Pocket Guide* in order to find full menus, plus shopping lists and menu substitutions for different dietary restrictions.

4-Week Meal Plan: Sample Menu

BREAKFAST

Cranberry Hazelnut Cereal: Mix 1½ cups Kashi 7 Whole Grain Puffs (105), 1 cup fat-free milk (80), 2 tablespoons **hazelnuts** (110), and 2 tablespoons dried cranberries (45). Have 1 medium orange (62). Total calories: 402.

LUNCH

Red Pepper Tapenade Wrap: Spread 1 whole wheat wrap (140) with 2 tablespoons **black olive tapenade** (88) and fill with ⅓ cup roasted red peppers (12). Have 1 cup fat-free milk (80) and 1 medium orange (62). Total calories: 382.

SNACK

Hummus Dip: Dip 1 cup sliced red bell peppers (46) into ½ cup hummus (200) sprinkled with 2 tablespoons **pine nuts** (113). Total calories: 359.

DINNER

Baby Green Pocket: Fill 1 whole wheat pita (140) with a mixture of 1 cooked and crumbled veggie burger (100), 1 cup mixed baby greens (9), ½ cup cooked corn (66), and 2 tablespoons **pecans**. Total calories: 405.

From the Flat Belly Diet! Pocket Guide

- Select **whole fruits and vegetables** over canned goods. Chop them into smaller sizes when you get home from the store and keep them in the refrigerator so that they're ready at snack time.

- Check canned or dried fruits and vegetables for added sugar, fat, or salt.

- Organic fruits and vegetables are lower in contaminants and healthier for the environment. Going organic is especially important with the Environmental Working Group's "dirty dozen" fruits and vegetables: peaches, apples, bell peppers, celery, nectarines, strawberries, cherries, lettuce, imported grapes, pears, spinach, and potatoes.

- When buying frozen or dried starchy vegetables, be sure to buy products with little or no added salt, and rinse them well before use.

- Today's supermarkets have a variety of fruits and vegetables that would have stunned our grandparents. If you're the kind of person who worries that dieting will limit your food options, change around the fruit and vegetable ingredients in your recipes to have an endless variety.

Whole Grains

Get your carbohydrates from unprocessed grains that have not had their fiber-rich bran and germ removed. You'll get much more fiber, nutrients, antioxidants, and phytochemicals that way.

- **100-percent whole grain** products, containing no refined flours, are your best friends here. Bread, cereals, couscous, rice, crackers, and pasta can all be made from 100-percent whole grains.

- Amaranth, barley, brown rice, buckwheat, bulgur wheat, cracked wheat, millet, oats, popcorn, quinoa, rye, spelt, whole wheat, and wild rice are all popular **whole grains** to look for in ingredient lists.

- **Avoid** enriched wheat flour (both bleached and unbleached), cornmeal, rice flour, semolina or durum flour, white flour, and white rice.

- Carb-bashing is in fashion, but if you follow the Flat Belly Diet! recipes, you'll get plenty of healthy carbs. The real carb villains are refined grains and sugary foods like candy, cookies, cakes, and sodas—those should be in your diet sparingly.

A Flat Belly Diet! Sample Shopping Trip

The Flat Belly Diet! contains four shopping lists, one for every week of the 4-Week Meal Plan. Here's the list from Week 1 to give you an idea of what you're going to be eating:

WEEK 1 SHOPPING LIST

PRODUCE

- Apples, any type, 8 medium (using 8)
- Granny Smith apples, 2 medium (using 2)
- Bananas, 5 small (using 5)
- Grapefruit, 3 (using 3)
- Mangoes, 2 fresh or frozen unsweetened chunks, 10-ounce bag (using 10 ounces)
- Strawberries, 18 ounces fresh or frozen unsweetened, 2 (10-ounce) packages (using $3\frac{1}{2}$ cups or 18 ounces)
- Hass avocados, 4 small (using 4)
- Baby carrots, 4-ounce package (1 cup) (using 1 cup)
- Cucumber, 1 small (using 1)
- Romaine lettuce, 3 (10-ounce) packages (using 3 packages)
- Red bell peppers, 3 medium (using 3)
- Tomatoes, 7 small (using 7)
- Orange juice, 100% pure, 1 quart
- Cilantro, 1 small bunch fresh (optional) (using 1)
- Parsley, 1 small bunch fresh (optional) (using 1)
- Tarragon, 1 small bunch fresh (optional) (using 1)

DAIRY

- Fat-free milk, $\frac{1}{2}$ gallon (using 5 cups)
- Laughing Cow Light Garlic & Herb Wedges, 6-ounce package (using 5 wedges)

- String cheese, 6-ounce package light or low-fat (using 3 pieces)* (If you are starting this plan immediately after doing the 4-Day Jump Start, you should have 2 pieces string cheese left over to use this week.)

EGGS

- Liquid egg whites, 8-ounce container (using ½ cup)

FROZEN FOODS

- Whole grain frozen waffles, 1 package (using 6)

- Whole cut corn, no salt added, 10-ounce package frozen

- Edamame (soybeans), 2 (10-ounce) packages frozen shelled

- Stir-fry or Chinese-style frozen vegetables (may include broccoli, carrots, cauliflower, mushrooms, water chestnuts; but if this mixture is not available, select a similar mixture), 2 (10-ounce) packages

- Meatless chicken-style nuggets, 2 (12-ounce) boxes

- Veggie burgers, 2 (4-count) packages, (using 2)

BREAD/CEREAL

- Whole wheat bread, 1-pound loaf, 16 slices (using 4 slices)

- Whole wheat pita pockets, about 6" diameter, 1 (8-count) package (using 7)

- Whole wheat wraps, 8" diameter, 1 (6-count) package

- Whole wheat crackers, about 1½" square, 12-ounce box (using 42)

- Rolled oats, 18-ounce canister

- Kashi 7 Whole Grain Puffs, 12-ounce box (using 2 cups)

DRY GOODS

- Canola oil, 8-ounce bottle

- Flaxseed oil, 8-ounce bottle cold-pressed (If you are starting this plan immediately after doing the 4-Day Jump Start, you should have enough

*We call for light or low-fat string cheese rather than part-skim because it is lower in saturated fat and calories. If you have trouble finding light or low-fat string cheese, though, feel free to substitute with part-skim string cheese.

flaxseed oil to take you through the 28-day plan and don't need to buy any more.)

- Extra virgin olive oil, 8-ounce bottle (using 3 tablespoons plus 1 teaspoon) (If you are starting this plan immediately after doing the 4-Day Jump Start, you should have enough olive oil to take you through the 28-day plan and don't need to buy more.)

- High-oleic safflower oil, 8-ounce bottle

- Sesame oil, 6-ounce bottle

- Sunflower oil, 8-ounce bottle

- Almond butter, 8-ounce jar (using 10 tablespoons)

- Almonds, 8-ounce package roasted or raw unsalted

- Brazil nuts, 6-ounce package roasted or raw unsalted

- Hazelnuts, ¼ cup bulk (or 2-ounce package) raw or roasted unsalted

- Macadamia nuts, ¼ cup bulk (or 2-ounce package) raw unsalted

- Pecans, 1 cup bulk (or 8-ounce package) roasted or raw unsalted

- Pine nuts, 6-ounce package roasted or raw unsalted

- Pistachios, ½ cup bulk (or 4-ounce package) raw unsalted

- Walnut halves, 6-ounce package raw unsalted (using 14 tablespoons)

- Peanut butter, natural, 12-ounce jar

- Peanuts, ⅛ cup bulk (or 2-ounce package), roasted or raw unsalted (using 2 tablespoons)

- Pumpkin seeds, ½ cup bulk (or 8-ounce package), roasted or raw unsalted (using 6 tablespoons)

- Sesame seeds, 2 tablespoons or ¾ ounce

- Sunflower seeds, ½ cup bulk (or 3-ounce package) raw unsalted

- Cannellini beans, no salt added, 15-ounce can

- Kidney beans, no salt added, 15-ounce can

- Green olives, 15-ounce jar large

- Black olives, 15-ounce can plus 7-ounce can large

- Semisweet or dark chocolate chips, 12-ounce package (using ½ cup)

- Cranberries, dried, unsweetened, 8-ounce package

- Raisins, seedless, 15-ounce container (If you are starting this plan immediately after doing the 4-Day Jump Start, you should have enough raisins to take you through the 28-day plan and don't need to buy any more.)

- Pineapple tidbits, packed in juice, 20-ounce can plus 8-ounce can (or eight 4-ounce cups) (using 4 ounces)

- Roasted red peppers, 12-ounce jar

- Dijon mustard, 8-ounce or smaller jar (using 4 teaspoons)

- Canola oil mayonnaise, 8-ounce jar

- Agave nectar, 1 small bottle (using 4 teaspoons)

- Chicken broth, reduced-sodium, 2 (16-ounce) cans

- Marinara sauce with less than 400 milligrams of sodium per ½-cup serving, 8-ounce jar

MEAL REPLACEMENT BARS

- Choose 7 of any of the following meal replacement bars. These bars are interchangeable on the plan wherever you see a bar listed with a meal or snack.

- Luna: Chai Tea, Chocolate Pecan Pie, or Lemon Zest Bar

- Nature's Path: Optimum Energy Bar Blueberry Flax & Soy or Pomegran Cherry

MEAT/SEAFOOD

- Wild salmon, 6-ounce can, or 8 ounces fresh salmon (using 6 ounces) (If you prefer to bake or broil your own salmon for these meals, purchase 3 ounces raw salmon for each 2 ounces cooked salmon in your meals. The raw weight for fish and meat is a little more than the cooked weight.)

- Chunk light water-pack tuna, 4 (3-ounce) cans (or two 6-ounce cans) or fresh or frozen tuna steak, 14 ounces (divide into 3½-ounce portions, store in freezer, defrost, and cook as needed)

• Organic deli chicken breast, 12-ounce package (using 12 ounces)**

SPICES AND SEASONINGS

- Ginger, ground, 1-ounce container
- Basil, dried, 1-ounce container
- Balsamic vinegar, aged, 8-ounce bottle (using 4 tablespoons)
- Rice vinegar, 6-ounce bottle (using 2 tablespoons)
- Sherry vinegar, 6-ounce bottle

SUBSTITUTIONS

A few commonsense substitutions can change the way you stock your pantry. Here are a few examples of products you can put in your shopping cart and others you can leave behind:

- Instead of butter or stick margarine, buy MUFA-rich spreads such as avocados or hummus.
- Instead of regular peanut butter, buy all-natural peanut, almond, or cashew butter.
- Instead of white, processed pasta, buy whole wheat or whole grain pasta.
- Instead of high-sodium bottled dressings and marinades, buy MUFA-rich olive oil and mix with balsamic or rice vinegar.

Flat Belly Diet! Pocket Guide contains more quick, easy shopping-cart substitutions. As a good rule of thumb, buy whole foods instead of processed foods, low- or zero-fat alternatives to high-fat ingredients, and snacks without additional sweetening. Dried fruit is a good example of a food that contains enough natural sweetness that you don't need to buy the varieties with added sweeteners, even if they contain natural sugars.

And go back to the basics when you can spare the time. The salad dressing substitution in the list above is a great example of a way you can strip out unnecessary additives from your life and improve your meals and your health at the same time.

**We call for organic deli meat because it is generally lower in sodium and fat. If you choose to purchase nonorganic meat, please look for low-sodium choices.

Living in the Real World

Let's face it: There's never a perfect time to try a new diet or exercise program. I know that, and so do Liz Vaccariello and Cynthia Sass, the authors of the *Flat Belly Diet!*. Just like the 4-Week Workout in Chapter 7 has a specific plan with a list of poses for every day of the week, Vaccariello and Sass's book contains specific daily meal plans for every day of the 4-Week Meal Plan. And similar to the tips and tricks that I included in Chapter 8, the Flat Belly Diet! also recognizes that in our busy lives, we are not often going to have 28 days in a row where everything we do is under our complete control. So take a look at how the Flat Belly Diet! is flexible and accommodates our busy lives.

It's easy to **swap MUFAs.** All of a sudden, if you're not in the mood for the next meal on the list, just make sure that when you improvise your replacement

mat motivation

Eat, Play, Love

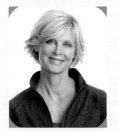

Okay, let's be straight with each other: Watching what we eat is one of the hardest things to do in life. Human beings are animals, and animals sometimes have strong cravings.

I have a weakness for chocolate chip cookies, and my students like to test my willpower by bringing me every variety known to mankind (I fail the test nearly every time). We all have foods we can't resist, and sweets are my downfall. So how do I control my sweets addiction? Well, it's pretty simple—I don't keep them in the house. (If I did, they wouldn't last very long anyway.)

Now, this isn't always a perfect solution. You may have a partner who loves to have a lot of food in the house, like I do. (Think muffins, lemonade, chips—you name it.)

Here's the great equalizer: Flat Belly Yoga!. Because I work out almost every day, I can indulge. Don't get me wrong—I don't binge on pizza and potato chips every day. I'm actually a pretty healthy eater, and from time to time I'll even do a juice cleanse.

But I enjoy my life, and that includes eating what I want sometimes, without the guilt. It's all about balance—and that balance is a lot easier to achieve if you're doing the Flat Belly Yoga! Workout because you'll be burning off those calories.

meal, you're getting the same amount of calories from MUFAs. For example, a 100-MUFA-calorie meal might have ¼ cup of Hass avocado. So swap this out for the same amount of calories, which can be found in 2 tablespoons of cashews, or in 1 tablespoon of pesto sauce plus ½ tablespoon of walnuts. You can also swap meals around—all you have to do is make sure that you get the same amount of total calories and MUFA calories every day. Then you can mix and match from the list of recipes until your heart (or your stomach) is content.

Many **store brands** are approved for use in the Flat Belly Diet!. Shop for Earth Balance Natural Almond Butter, Cantaré Olive Tapenade, Dagoba Organic Sweet Dark Chocolate Bars, or Polly-O String Cheese. There are even prepackaged meals that fit easily into the diet. Combine Amy's Kitchen Organic Brown Rice, Black Eyed Peas & Veggies Bowl with 2 tablespoons of peanuts for an easy 400-calorie dinner. Or add 2 tablespoons of MUFA-rich pumpkin seeds to Kashi Southwest Style Chicken for an easy meal with a gourmet flavor.

But what if you're out at a **restaurant**? The Flat Belly Diet! has plenty of suggestions for national brands as well as typical independent restaurants. For example, at Chipotle, you can order two 6" Tortilla Wraps, top with Pinto Beans, lettuce and salsa, and add 2 tablespoons of pistachios to create a MUFA-rich, 418-calorie meal. At any Italian trattoria, you can order cooked whole wheat pasta, and combine 1 cup of the pasta with ½ tablespoon olive oil, 1 tablespoon Parmesan cheese, and flavor with black pepper. Then have a side salad dressed with another ½ tablespoon olive oil and a splash of vinegar. Add either ¾ cup minestrone soup or a 2-ounce portion of broiled salmon.

One tip that works just about anywhere you go: Carry your own tablespoon! It will make your life easier in two ways. First, you won't have to bag precise measurements of nuts and seeds or other foods to take with you. Second, when you're out at a restaurant or a friend's house, you won't have to ask them to measure food amounts. You can get a small ramekin or side dish of pumpkin seeds, peanuts, or even avocado and measure it yourself to make sure your portions are precise and filling. (And it's especially easy when you're whipping up your own salad dressing tableside.)

The Flat Belly Diet! also features a wide variety of diet substitutes for vegan, vegetarian, and gluten- and soy-free diets. Not only are all of the basic

MUFA-rich foods included in each of those diets, but many specially prepared substitutes fit right into the Flat Belly Diet! Vegan meat alternatives such as Tofurky Deli Slices and Rice Dream Rice Milk, soy-free staples such as Horizon Organic Cheddar Slices or Kashi 7 Whole Grain Puffs, dairy-free items like Tofutti soy cheese and Luna Bar snacks, and gluten-free foods such as Health Valley unsweetened cornflakes and Applegate Farms turkey are allowed.

You Can Do It

Combining your Flat Belly Yoga! Workout with the Flat Belly Diet! Meal Plan will make you feel stronger and more energized. You'll have a greater sense of control over your health and how you feel and look.

A 1,600-calorie plan—built around consistent 400-calories meals that are based on MUFAs and make smart use of lean proteins, whole grains, and fruits and vegetables—is a sustainable diet. Not only will it help you reach your weight loss goals, but as you incorporate its principles into your daily nutrition plan, it will also help you keep the weight off for good.

PLAY IT SAFE Don't use food as a reward! Did you walk an extra 10 minutes or stick to your diet today? Don't "reward" yourself with that cupcake you saw in the bakery window. Remember: Your reward is how great you'll look and feel.

A FLAT BELLY YOGA SUCCESS STORY

Laura Prabucki Calandra

Age: 34

Pounds lost:

10

in 32 days

All-over inches lost:

9.5

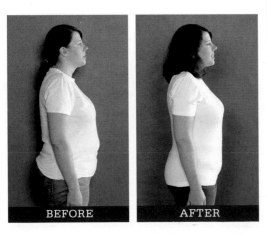

BEFORE   AFTER

"My upcoming wedding was my motivation to safely lose weight that would stay off," says Laura Prabucki Calandra. Having practiced yoga for the last 3 years, she knew firsthand the physical and mental benefits that yoga could provide. But Laura also knew she needed something more to meet her goal.

After committing to the Flat Belly Yoga! program, Laura wasn't surprised by how much she enjoyed the workouts. "My favorite part of the program was the yoga with weights portion," she says. "I love a challenge and knew that adding weights to my yoga routine would challenge me both mentally and physically. I knew that this program would take my yoga practice to the next level."

What did come as a surprise, however, was how much she loved the diet. Before trying the Flat Belly Diet!, Laura says her meals left her feeling deprived. "I ate moderately healthy, but was limiting my carbohydrates and occasionally making myself miserable. The Flat Belly Diet! was simple, yet tasty—and you can have carbs and dairy!"

Laura found that the Flat Belly Diet! meal plans were easy to follow—and most of the ingredients she needed to prepare her meals were already stocked in her kitchen. In fact, the diet was so simple and flexible that the 34-year-old says she has now completely changed her way of eating.

"I am incorporating this meal plan into

my everyday life. I am now more conscious of what I'm eating—especially while on the road, as I travel a lot for work," she says. "With a few simple swaps, I can still eat the foods I like. I also found that if there is a MUFA I don't like, I can swap it for something else."

And the best part of the diet for Laura? It didn't leave her feeling hungry or fatigued. "The diet and workouts definitely go hand-in-hand," she describes. "The food provided me with enough energy to get through the workouts. As you are losing belly fat by eating healthy foods, you are also tightening your core through the Flat Belly Yoga! poses. With the diet and the yoga, those unwanted inches go away quickly!"

After the first full week of the program, Laura says she felt less bloated. She was also sleeping better, had more energy, and noticed more tone in her arms and belly with each passing week.

Having lost most of the inches from her waist and thighs, Laura knew she had accomplished the goal she set for herself 4 weeks earlier. "In the past, I didn't think it was possible to lose inches that quickly, and it is," she exclaims. "It was such a great feeling having my wedding dress taken in several times as the weight came off. I was so excited to begin my new life with my husband and my new figure. It's always nice to have people tell you 'you look great' and know they actually mean it!

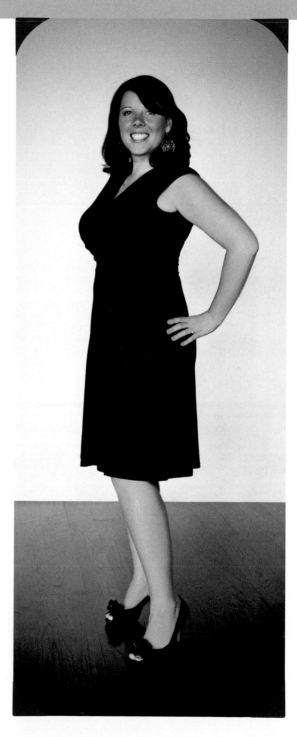

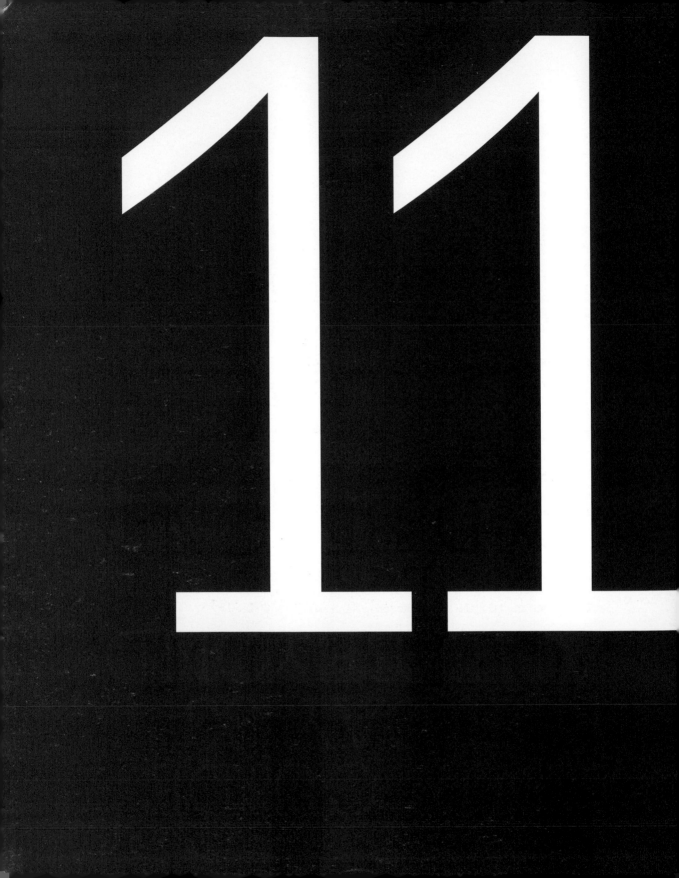

YOUR GUIDE FOR DAY 33 AND BEYOND

If you're reading this chapter, one of two things has happened:

Option 1: You may have been so interested in what you've seen in *Flat Belly Yoga!* that you've read through the whole book, including the 4-Day Jump Start and the 4-Week Workout, and you've decided that you can do it.

If that's the case, congratulations! Because I know you're right. You *can* do it. And by reading this far, you've strengthened your chances of successfully achieving your goal of getting the flat belly you've always wanted.

You now know what yoga can do for you, especially when you add weights and combine it with cardio. You also know how to get yourself off the couch with the Jump Start, *and* you've read about what your whole month will look like. So there should be no surprises in store for you!

You have a number of tips and tricks at your disposal that you can use to keep yourself motivated, including your journal, the single most important motivational tool you can have.

So here's an important decision for you to make (if you haven't already): Are you going to use the Flat Belly Diet! program with your workout? You know about all the delicious options that are available in a MUFA-rich, scientifically supported nutrition program. Hopefully you're thinking that you might just be ambitious enough to combine the diet with your workouts. And why not? It's a great goal because the two programs were designed to be used together.

As they say, knowledge is power. Right now, you are ready to start exercising (and possibly dieting). You are ready to take on that frustrating problem area and significantly improve your health by doing so. And you are ready to change your life. It sounds like a tall order. But if you've read this far, you have an advantage over everyone else who wonders, day after day, whether they can get in shape. You *know* you can do it.

So what are you waiting for? Put on your exercise clothes, go to your chosen space, and do your first Jump Start workout today! This chapter will still be here when you get back.

Option 2: So maybe you decided you didn't need to read the whole book in order to get started. Maybe you've finished the whole Flat Belly Yoga! 32-day program. If that's the case, then *congratulations!* I am very proud of you. You did it! But you don't need me to tell you that. You're proud of yourself, right? You should be.

I'm sure that after completing the program, you're looking better in your jeans. You're sleeping better. You have more energy. And you feel all-around great about yourself. But don't go putting this book down just quite yet. You don't think that you and I are finished with each other, do you?

Because as happy as I am that you got this far, I have something else in mind for you. You've been concentrating on one month of your life. Well, I've been thinking about the big picture. I want you to stay happy with your health and your body (especially your belly) for the rest of your life.

So like any good coach, I'm not going to let up just yet. I'm going to keep on top of you. I am not willing to allow you to let yourself down.

Keep Moving

The Web site HealthyPeople.gov provides "science-based, 10-year objectives for improving the health of all Americans." Their Physical Activity Guidelines set standards for exercise and activity that all of us should be able to easily meet. But according to the most recent statistics, most Americans don't meet them. Only 20.4 percent of adults 18 years of age and over meet those guidelines for both aerobic and muscle-strengthening physical activity.[1]

So guess what? Right now, knowing nothing else about you besides the fact that you completed the Flat Belly Yoga! program, I can tell you this much: You are in the top 20 percent of active Americans. (Probably higher.) Right now, you are not down in the dumps with four-fifths of all Americans who don't get the physical activity they need. Quite the opposite! Now you're part of the healthy, active elite. If you continue to incorporate the tools I've given you into your everyday life, you can keep counting yourself among the 20 percent of Americans who meet the guidelines. You've got your muscle-strengthening activity in the Core+Yoga routines and your aerobic exercise in the form of Heart Walks.

But if you're anything like me, my guess is that you're not getting a whole lot of personal validation from simply beating the government statistics, right? If you've completed the 32 days of the Flat Belly Yoga! Workout, I bet you feel and look great—and I'm willing to go out on a limb and say you want to *continue* feeling and looking great.

Weight loss is great. A flat belly is something to be proud of. But you want to know a secret (that's not so secret)? The other benefits of exercise can be life changing.

A FLAT BELLY YOGA
SUCCESS STORY

Shari Robins

Age: 49

Pounds lost:
11
in 32 days

All-over inches lost:
14.5

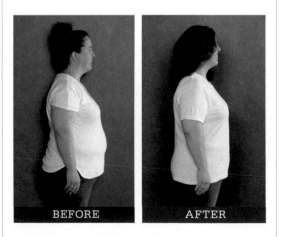

BEFORE   AFTER

"I had ballooned to 209 pounds and needed something to kick-start my weight loss," states Shari Robins. As a chef, Shari struggled to keep her weight down. Part of her job was developing high-carb products, such as pancakes, cupcakes, cookies, stuffing, rice, and pasta, for a major grocery chain. She also was dealing with a number of physical issues, including two knee surgeries and back surgery. But Shari knew she could lose weight because she had done it before.

During the 32-day program, she went down from a size 16-18 to a size 14-16. "The good news is that I have jeans in all sizes—from an 18 all the way down to a 6, which I look forward to fitting into," she says. "I have lost large amounts of weight several times in my life, and as I enter my fiftieth year, I think to myself, *How many more times do you want to lose and gain weight?* My answer is zero. This is my last."

Shari knew that losing the weight would not be easy and that it would take a lot of commitment and focus. She also knew that finding the time to exercise would be the biggest challenge. She went from literally doing no exercise during the last few years to exercising 6 days per week. "I learned that I have the strength to do anything I set my mind to. I learned—or rather, remembered—that I like to exercise. And I was tired of carrying around an extra 70 pounds."

Once Shari decided to combine the Flat Belly Yoga! program with the Flat Belly Diet! to achieve optimal results, she found that the diet offered just the variety she wanted. "I loved the diet and loved my food options," she says. "I was able to interchange ingredients from the different recipes to work for my palate. Eating has always been complicated for me because it is part of my job. I have to eat out, check out new chefs, and be on top of the latest food trends. In addition, I often feel pressured to cook something creative and reinvent the wheel." During the program, she learned to tell herself that every meal didn't need to be gourmet and over-the-top as long as it was healthy and satisfying.

It wasn't always easy, but the more she got into the program, the more excited she was to lose the weight and get in shape. After the 4-Day Jump Start and the first week of the plan, her friends and family immediately noticed that she looked healthier. "I felt good after the first week. In addition to the weight loss, I also noticed that I was sleeping better," she explains. "During the second and third weeks, I started to notice my energy level increasing."

And Shari knows that continuing to follow the program will help her fight the temptation she faces at work—stating that she wants to take the Flat Belly Yoga! plan to Day 33—and beyond! "I enjoyed the regimen of it all—regular yoga practice, regular walking, and a regular eating routine," she says. "I do well with a set program like this, so I felt I could continue to follow this plan even after the 32 days were over. I will never be done with this 'program'—it will become my new way of life! "

Now that you're riding high on your accomplishment, it's the perfect time to step back and look at the big picture. Remembering that regular exercise changes your whole life for the better makes it a little easier to continue your Flat Belly Yoga! Workout beyond the last day of the plan.

But in case you need a better motivator than just looking good in your skinny jeans, consider these reasons to get—and keep—moving:

Exercise helps build and maintain immunity. Workouts raise your body temperature, strengthening the immune system over time. They may also reduce the risk of breast and prostate cancers by regulating hormone levels. Exercise to the point of exhaustion isn't recommended when you're sick, but research consistently shows that people who exercise frequently have a much higher resistance to colds and other communicable diseases than more sedentary people.[2]

Exercise protects your heart. Getting the heart pumping works wonders for decreasing the risk factors associated with heart attacks. It strengthens the heart muscle, makes the heart more efficient, improves the flow of blood to the heart muscle, and—one of the most valuable effects of all—improves the heart's ability to handle stress. If you continue this program, you'll even raise your good cholesterol (HDL), lower your blood pressure, and reduce arterial inflammation.

Exercise balances your blood sugar. This is especially true if you break a sweat. (And if you're not breaking a sweat, you might want to go back and read the section on interval training again. Remember my coach from Chapter 6? "Pick it up!") A regular sweat can decrease your risk of type 2 diabetes by increasing sensitivity to insulin—not to mention by helping to manage your weight. In fact, a study published in the medical journal *Annals of Internal Medicine* found that you can reduce your risk of type 2 diabetes by 34 percent simply by taking a brisk walk for one hour daily.[3]

Exercise lifts your mood. Remember when I talked about the mood-changing wonders of exercise in Chapter 4? The ability of endorphins to change your mood is a whole lot more than a flash-in-the-pan effect. Regular aerobic exercise has been shown to be as effective as medication in relieving depression.

A study undertaken by researchers at the University of Rochester Medical Center in New York found that people undergoing treatment for depression had just as good results with exercise as people taking selective serotonin reuptake inhibitors (SSRIs) like Prozac or Lexapro. And in some cases, the exercisers had better results.[4]

Another study found that an exercise program was an effective replacement for "second treatment" prescriptions such as lithium.[5] Note: If you receive medical treatment to help you deal with depression, you should talk with your doctor before replacing your prescriptions with an exercise program.

Exercise helps manage menopause. Exercises like walking and yoga elevate your mood and help manage the symptoms of menopause. Some research indicates that estrogen levels rise after exercise, helping to decrease the severity of hot flashes. A study that appeared in the *Journal of Advanced Nursing* showed significant improvement in the conditions of a group of menopausal women between the ages of 55 and 72 who participated in a fully supervised exercise program three times a week for 12 months. The study also reported that the participants' overall quality of life improved as well.[6]

Exercise makes you look younger. Enough said, right? Aerobic activity like your Heart Walk increases oxygen consumption during exercise, which can take years off your appearance and even stimulate new brain cells. Remember when we talked about *sarcopenia* (the phenomenon of losing muscle mass as we age) in Chapter 2? Researchers at Tel Aviv University recently discovered that exercise activates the stem cells in our muscles—creating new tissue from the ground up in ways that defy what we thought we knew about the irreversibility of aging.[7]

And there are other fountain-of-youth effects from exercise that we've known about for a while and medical science is just starting to verify. For example, your cells contain telomeres that act as biological clocks—they wind down as you age, similar to a pocket watch ticking slowly to a halt. However, they don't wind down very quickly if you commit to a program of regular exercise.

In 2009, the journal *Circulation* published research showing that middle-aged runners had telomeres that resembled those of 20-year-olds. By getting

Life and Nothing But

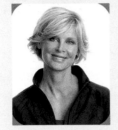

At the beginning of your journey, you were probably thinking: I don't know if I can commit to 32 days. But you did, right? Well, now I want you to commit even longer—for the rest of your life!

I know that seems hard—and maybe even impossible. But think about how good you feel now. Don't you want to hang onto this feeling forever? Well, you can!

I learned this at an early age, thanks mostly to my dad. He was hoping for a boy, but that didn't stop him from taking me with him to judo lessons when I was 3 years old. This was the beginning of my love of fitness. And it wasn't long before I had the confidence to flip a kid in my kindergarten class who kept pulling my ponytail. I got suspended, but he never touched me again.

So here's my point: We are happier, healthier, and more confident when we're in shape. And that's the best incentive for maintaining a workout regimen over the long haul. Still not convinced? Well, let's make a list of the benefits and downsides of regular exercise.

PLUSES

- Energizes you for the day
- Slims and strengthens your body
- Builds your self-esteem
- Improves your overall health
- Enhances your sex life
- Clears your mind
- Rids you of angst
- Helps you sleep better
- Takes off excess weight
- Allows you to eat what you want (well, at least more than you could if you didn't work out)

MINUSES

- Takes time (but only in the short term because exercising regularly can extend your life by several years)

Now I want you to look back over this list and try to add a few pluses of your own. And I'll bet you a chocolate chip cookie that there won't be any more minuses.

your heart rate up, you pump blood throughout your body—through your veins, arteries, and the capillaries that run underneath your skin. This has strong detoxifying effects, not to mention rejuvenating effects on your appearance.[8]

Exercise lets you live longer. A 2007 study in the *Journal of the American Medical Association* found that fitter people lived longer, even if they had extra pounds around the middle.[9] Among 2,603 adults age 60 and older enrolled in that longitudinal study, the fittest people (those who did best on a treadmill test) also had the lowest risk factors for hypertension, diabetes, and high cholesterol. That should make you want to continue to lace up your walking shoes!

Flat Belly for Life: Rules to Make You Move

I can't write out an exercise program for you for every day of the rest of your life. And I shouldn't have to. With the exercise routines and the tips and tricks you've learned in *Flat Belly Yoga!*, you should have everything you need to make exercise a permanent part of your daily life.

Life's going to throw obstacles in front of you. Did you take your copy of *Flat Belly Yoga!* with you to a tropical island with no one around for 32 days? My guess is, no, you didn't—which means that you've already had to protect your exercise time from family, friends, errands, emergencies, and "emergencies." (And you know what? Even if you could take 32 days in paradise, I bet there would be a day when you *just didn't feel like exercising*.)

There are too many forces lined up against us to be perfect exercisers. But we don't have to be perfect exercisers—we have to be good exercisers. Most importantly, we have to enjoy exercise—both the short-term benefits of having time to ourselves and doing physical activity, and the longer-term benefits for our health and our looks.

I'm going to break it down for you into three simple rules. If you can make these three rules a permanent part of your life, you're going to have no problem getting and keeping the belly you want.

- Rule 1: Move 6 days a week.
- Rule 2: Weigh yourself every day.
- Rule 3: Keep journaling.

Rule 1: MOVE 6 DAYS A WEEK.

Now that you've completed the Flat Belly Yoga! program, I'm hoping you're feeling like you've set a bar for yourself—and not like you've finished all the exercise you need to do. You might even want to bump it up because of just how good you feel. Ask yourself: How can you take your walking to the next level? You could try jogging or running.

Maybe you'd like to help raise money for charity by signing up for a charity race. You probably know people who have raised money for a cause or a cure by walking or running in a charity event. At my YAS Fitness Centers in Southern California, we host annual events that raise hundreds of thousands of dollars to fight cancer for ThinkCure!, a local community-based non-profit that raises funds for cancer research. And it's all done by individuals who step up and challenge themselves to beat their personal bests. How proud would you be if one of the effects of getting yourself off the couch and eliminating your belly fat was that you could raise hundreds or thousands of dollars for charity? That's getting more out of your skinny jeans than I bet you ever imagined!

Here are a few charity walks that may have local events near you:

The American Cancer Society sponsors the **Relay for Life**. www.relayforlife.org

The **Avon Walk for Breast Cancer** supports critical research and makes sure that brease cancer patients get the care they need. www.avonwalk.org

The Leukemia & Lymphoma Society sponsors the **Light the Night Walk** to raise money for people battling blood cancers. www.lightthenight.org

The National Kidney Foundation sponsors walks to raise money and awareness about kidney diseases and the need for organ donation. walk.kidney.org

Depending on where you live, you may be able to find a different walking event every weekend. Check the calendar section in your local newspaper. Or is there a cause you want to raise money for that doesn't have a walk? Connect with the organization to ask about hosting one. Large-scale charity walks are put on by companies in exchange for a percentage of the funds raised, but in your community you can probably put one together on a budget. Just make sure that most of the funds you raise go to the cause of your choice. You can even find instructions online about how to put together a charity walk. (But don't spend all your time planning—the point is to keep walking!)

Rule 2: WEIGH YOURSELF EVERY DAY.

We talked about this in Chapter 6 and I want to mention it again to emphasize its importance. (At the time, you were probably skimming because you were so eager to get to the workout, right?) If you can make daily observations of your weight as routine as brushing your teeth, it will give your weight less power over you—and it will give you more power over your weight. Weighing yourself whenever you feel like it is a recipe for anxious weighing, and you learned about the vicious circle of anxiety and stress in Chapter 4. Do it every day, and you'll become a scientist in your own laboratory. You have a steady stream of information, and that information is power. The alternative is being afraid of the information because you won't like what it says about you, which isn't helping you reach your goal.

By knowing what's going on "in the lab," you can make the adjustments you need to stay one step ahead of the weight gain. You can change up—or bump up—your exercise routine. You can give yourself the evidence you need to convince yourself to commit and recommit.

If you find that your belly or your weight isn't budging, then continue your Flat Belly Yoga! Workout and couple it with the Flat Belly Diet!. (Make sure to dial back your daily workout if you start with the calorie-restricted 4-Day Anti-Bloat Jump Start.)

It might sound like a lot, but you'll get the results you've been looking for. You might even want to try this combo again around the same time that you're getting ready for a big event. It might be a good idea if you have something special planned. Maybe it's your high school reunion. Maybe it's your big 50th birthday party. It's always good to have a goal and it's even better to have a deadline for that goal, whether it's something as big as a reunion or as small as an office party.

And here's one thing you can't forget: When you hit a goal with your weight, you have to reward yourself. (Don't reward yourself with food. That sets an unhealthy cycle of denial and indulgence, and it will create patterns that in the long run will defeat you in your belly battle.) Personally, I like to reward myself with a facial. There's nothing more relaxing to me than a soothing facial at a spa, especially after I've achieved a personal goal that I've struggled with. So choose a reward that means something to you and take the time to enjoy it.

Rule 3: KEEP JOURNALING.

In Chapter 9, we discussed the big advantage of keeping a daily journal. Writing down your thoughts and experience of working out will give you the focus and perspective you need to achieve your flat belly. It will give you an outlet for the surprising emotions that may come up as you take control of your belly, your body, your health, and your life. And it will give you a place where no one is allowed to judge you—not even yourself—for the shape you're in or the things you want to accomplish.

You will give yourself an incredible gift by making sure you stay mindful of your daily activities. You might want to jot down what makes you crazy during the day. This will help you with your relationship to working out. As you read in Chapter 4, there is a strong connection between stress and gaining weight or belly fat. Writing in your journal will not only keep you focused, but it will also give you a great place to release your stress. If you find that you're winding yourself up by bringing up all your emotions in your journal, one good trick is to release all of your air in a quick, loud exhale. Combined with writing down your feelings and observations, it will make stress an obstacle you can hop right over.

Stay Inspired

Hopefully, you are inspired with your new flat belly, your extra energy, and your deeper, healthier sleep. Now I want you to stay inspired! Make sure you sign up online for flatbellyyoga.com. The Web site, a project of www.prevention.com, features additional resources beyond those included in this book.

In Closing

I hope I have provided you with all the tools you will need to keep your belly flat for life. Remember this: You aren't doing the Flat Belly Yoga! Workout for your romantic partner, for your children, for your neighbors or colleagues, or for your friends. You're not doing it to look like the women on TV or in fashion magazines. And you're not doing it to compete with anyone else. You're doing it for you! And you are worth it!

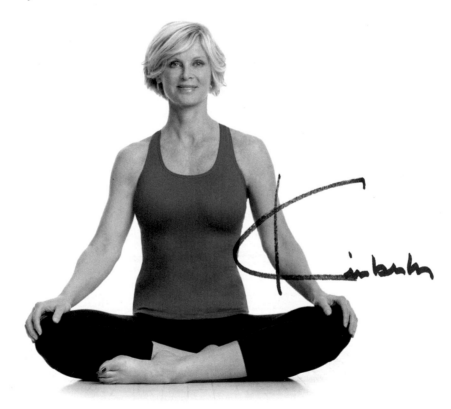

endnotes

Chapter 1

1. Anders, M. ACE yoga study: Does yoga really do the body good? *ACE Fitness Matters*. www.acefitness.org/getfit/studies/YogaStudy2005.pdf.

2. Yoga for anxiety and depression. *Harvard Mental Health Letter* (April 2009). Retrieved June 2012. www.health.harvard.edu/newsletters/Harvard_Mental_Health_Letter/2009/April/Yoga-for-anxiety-and-depression.

3. National Institutes of Health, National Institute of Neurological Disorders and Stroke (NINDS). Low back pain fact sheet. NIH publication no. 03-5161 (July 2003). www.ninds.nih.gov/disorders/backpain/detail_backpain.htm.

Chapter 2

1. Ryan, A. S., et al. Resistive training increases fat-free mass and maintains RMR despite weight loss in postmenopausal women. *Journal of Applied Physiology* 79, no. 3 (September 1, 1995): 818–23.

2. Canadian Science Publishing (NRC Research Press). Building muscle without heavy weights. *ScienceDaily* 26 (April 2012). Web. 7 Nov. 2012.

3. Ohkawa, S., Odamaki, M., Ikegaya, N., et al. Association of age with muscle mass, fat mass and fat distribution in non-diabetic haemodialysis patients. *Nephrology Dialysis Transplantation* 20, no. 5 (May 1, 2005): 945–51.

4. Abdominal fat and what to do about it. *Harvard Medical School Family Health Guide* (2007). www.health.harvard.edu/fhg/updates/Abdominal-fat-and-what-to-do-about-it.shtml.

5. Kravitz, L. Resistance training: Adaptations and health implications. *IDEA Today* 14, no. 9 (1996), 38–46. www.unm.edu/~lkravitz/Article%20folder/resistben.html.

6. Singh, N. A., Clements, K. M., and Fiatarone, M. A. A randomized controlled trial of the effect of exercise on sleep. *Sleep* 20, no. 2 (1997): 95–101.

7. Barnett, A., Smith, B., Lord, S., et al. Community-based group exercise improves balance and reduces falls in at-risk older people: A randomized controlled trial. *Age and Ageing* 32 (2003): 407–14.

8. O'Connor, P. J., Herring, M. P., and Carvalho, A. Mental health benefits of strength training in adults. *American Journal of Lifestyle Medicine* 4, no. 5 (2010): 377–96.

9. Ramirez, A., and Kravitz, L. Resistance training improves mental health. *IDEA Fitness Journal* 9, no. 1 (2012): 20–22.

10. Sigal, R. J., Kenny, G. P., Wasserman, D. H., Castaneda-Sceppa, C., and White, R. D. Physical activity/exercise and type 2 diabetes: A consensus statement from the American Diabetes Association. *Diabetes Care* 29, no. 6 (June 2006): 1433–8.

11. Kravitz, L. Yes, resistance training can reverse the aging process. *IDEA Fitness Journal* 5, no. 8 (2008): 21–23.

12. Westcott, W. L., and Loud, R. L. Fight cellulite. *Wellness.MA*, 2003. www.wellness.ma/diet/cellulite.htm.

Chapter 3

1. Slentz, C. A., et al. Effects of aerobic vs. resistance training on visceral and liver fat stores, liver enzymes, and insulin resistance by HOMA in overweight adults from STRRIDE AT/RT. *American Journal of Physiology–Endocrinology and Metabolism* 301 (2011): E1033–39.

2. Martina, Navratilova. Walking: The easiest exercise. *AARP* (September 29, 2010).

3. Mayo Clinic Staff. Walking: Trim your waistline, improve your health. Mayo Clinic (December 18, 2010). www.mayoclinic.com/health/walking/HQ01612.

4. Krall, E. A., and Dawson-Hughes, B. Walking is related to bone density and rates of bone loss. Calcium and Bone Metabolism Laboratory, U.S. Department of Agriculture Human Nutrition Research Center on Aging, Tufts University, Boston, Massachusetts.

5. Artal, M., and Sherman, C. Exercise against depression. *Physician and Sportsmedicine* 26, no. 10 (1998): 55–59.

6. Knubben, K., et al. A randomised, controlled study on the effects of a short-term endurance training programme in patients with major depression. *British Journal of Sports Medicine* 41, no. 1 (2007): 29–33.

7. Venturelli, M., Scarsini, R., and Schena, F. Six-month walking program changes cognitive and ADL performance in patients with Alzheimer's. *American Journal of Alzheimer's Disease and Other Dementias* (August 2011).

8. Berg, B. Morning exercise means a better night's sleep. Fred Hutchinson Cancer Research Center (December 4, 2003). www.fhcrc.org/en/news/center-news/2003/12/morning-exercise.html.

9. American College of Sports Medicine. *ACSM's Guidelines for Exercise and Prescription, 7th Edition.* Philadelphia: Lippincott Williams & Wilkins, 2005.

10. Allen, K., Blascovich, J., Tomaka, J., and Kelsey, R. Presence of human friends and pet dogs as moderators of autonomic responses to stress in women. *Journal of Personality and Social Psychology* 61 (1991), 582–89.

Chapter 4

1. Solberg Nes, L., and Segerstrom, S. C. The future of optimism. *American Psychologist* (2006).

2. Colin Jackson's raise your game: What are the benefits of listening to music? www.bbc.co.uk/wales/raiseyourgame/sites/motivation/psychedup/pages/costas_karageorghis.shtml.

3. Bouchez, C. Can stress cause weight gain?" *WebMD* (May 13, 2005). www.webmd.com/diet/features/can-stress-cause-weight-gain.

4. Epel, E. S., McEwen, B., Seeman, T., Matthews, K., Castellazzo, G., Brownell, K. D., Bell, J., and Ickovics, J. R. Stress and body shape: Stress-induced cortisol secretion is consistently greater among women with central fat. *Psychosomatic Medicine* 62, no. 5 (September-October 2000): 623–32.

5. Jennifer Daubenmier, Jean Kristeller, Frederick M. Hecht, Nicole Maninger, Margaret Kuwata, Kinnari Jhaveri, Robert H. Lustig, Margaret Kemeny, Lori Karan, and Elissa Epel. Mindfulness intervention for stress eating to reduce cortisol and abdominal fat among overweight and obese women: An exploratory randomized controlled study. *Journal of Obesity* (2011).

6. Martin, S. Our health at risk. *APA Monitor* 43, no. 18 (2012). www.apa.org/news/press/releases/stress/2011/health-risk.aspx.

7. Reynolds, G. Phys ed: Why exercise makes you less anxious. *New York Times Online* (November 18, 2009). www.well.blogs.nytimes.com/2009/11/18/phys-ed-why-exercise-makes-you-less-anxious.

8. Streeter, C. C., Whitfield, T. H., Owen, L., et al. Effects of yoga versus walking on mood, anxiety, and brain GABA levels: A randomized controlled MRS study. *Journal of Alternative and Complementary Medicine* 16, no. 11 (2010).

9. Paul, M. Aerobic exercise relieves insomnia. Northwestern University News Center (September 2010). www.northwestern.edu/newscenter/stories/2010/09/aerobic-exercise-relieves-insomnia.html.

10. Nedeltcheva, A. V., Kilkus, J. M., Imperial, J., et al. Insufficient sleep undermines dietary efforts to reduce adiposity. *Annals of Internal Medicine* 153, no. 7 (October 5, 2010): 435–41.

Chapter 5

1. Cohen, E., Ejsmond-Frey, R., Knight, N., and Dunbar, R. I. M. Rowers' high: Behavioural synchrony is correlated with elevated pain thresholds. *Biology Letters* 6 (2010): 106–108.

2. BMJ-British Medical Journal. Structured warm-up exercises may prevent up to half of severe sports injuries. *ScienceDaily* (December 22, 2008).

3. American College of Sports Medicine. Position stand on exercise and fluid replacement. *Medicine and Science in Sports and Exercise* 28, no. 1 (1996): i–vii.

Chapter 6

1. Gilchrist, J., Jones, B. H., Sleet, D. A., and Kimsey, C. D. Exercise-related injuries among women: Strategies for prevention from civilian and military studies. *MMWR Recommendations and Reports* 49, RR-2 (March 31 2000): 15–33.

2. Lee, J., et al. Effects of yoga exercise on serum adiponectin and metabolic syndrome factors in obese postmenopausal women. *Menopause* 19, no. 3 (March 2012): 296–301.

3. Leading Causes of Death for American Women. The Heart Truth. 2008. www.nhlbi.nih.gov/educational/hearttruth/downloads/html/infographic-dressgraph-bw/infograph1.htm.

4. Deaths: final data for 2008. *National Vital Statistics Reports* 59, no. 10 (December 7, 2011): 43–46.

5. CDC. Prevalence and most common causes of disability among adults–United States, 2005. *MMWR* 58, no. 16 (2009): 421–26.

6. NIH: National Heart, Lung, and Blood Institute.

7. Lindquist, R., Boucher, J. L., Grey, E. Z., et al. Eliminating untimely deaths of women with heart disease: Highlights from the Minnesota Women's Heart Summit. *American Heart Journal* 163, no. 1 (2012): A1–8.

Chapter 8

1. Bureau of Labor Statistics. American time use survey—2011 results. June 22, 2012.

2. Pope, E. Sitting: Hazardous to your health. *AARP Bulletin* (January-February 2012): 28–30.

3. Levine, J. A., Schleusner, S. J., Jensen, M. D. Energy expenditure of nonexercise activity. *American Journal of Clinical Nutrition* 72, no. 6 (December 2002): 1451–54.

4. Wen, C. P., Wai, J. P., Tsai, M. K., et al. Minimum amount of physical activity for reduced mortality and extended life expectancy: A prospective cohort study. *Lancet* 378, no. 9798 (2011): 1244–53.

5. Corliss, J. Lose weight and keep it off. *Harvard Health Publications.* 2011. www.health.harvard.edu/special_health_reports/lose-weight-and-keep-it-off.

6. Peetz, J., Buehler, R., and Britten, K. Only minutes a day: Reframing exercise duration affects exercise intentions and behavior. *Basic and Applied Social Psychology* 33, no. 2. (May 2011): 118–27.

Chapter 9

1. Smyth, J. M., Stone, A. A., Hurewitz, A., et al. Effects of writing about stressful experiences on symptom reduction in patients with asthma or rheumatoid arthritis: A randomized trial. *JAMA* 281, no. 14 (1999): 1304–09.

Chapter 11

1. Centers for Disease Control and Prevention. www.cdc.gov/nchs/fastats/exercise.htm.

2. Nieman, D. C. Moderate exercise improves immunity and decreases illness rates. *American Journal of Lifestyle Medicine* 5, no. 4 (July-August 2011): 338–45.

3. Hu, F. B., Stampfer, M. J., Solomon, C., et al. Physical activity and risk for cardiovascular events in diabetic women. *Annals of Internal Medicine* 134, no. 2 (January 2001): 96–105.

4. Rethorst, C. D., et al. Efficacy of exercise in reducing depressive symptoms across 5-HTTLPR genotypes. *Medicine and Science in Sports and Exercise* 42, no. 11 (November 2010): 2141–47.

5. Trivedi, M. H., Greer, T. L., Church, T. S., et al. Exercise as an augmentation treatment for nonremitted major depressive disorder: a randomized, parallel dose comparison. *Journal of Clinical Psychiatry* 72, no. 5 (May 2011): 677–84.

6. Villaverde-Gutiérrez, C., Araújo, E., Cruz, F., Roa, J. M., Barbosa, W., and Ruíz-Villaverde, G. Quality of life of rural menopausal women in response to a customized exercise programme. *Journal of Advanced Nursing* 54 (2006): 11–19.

7. Shefer, G., Rauner, G., Yablonka-Reuveni, Z., and Benayahu, D. Reduced satellite cell numbers and myogenic capacity in aging can be alleviated by endurance exercise. *PLoS ONE* 5, no. 10 (2010): e13307. doi:10.1371/journal.pone.0013307.

8. Werner, C., Fürster, T., Widmann, T., et al. Physical exercise prevents cellular senescence in circulating leukocytes and in the vessel wall. *Circulation* 120, no. 24 (December 15, 2009): 2438–47.

9. Sui, X., LaMonte, M. J., Laditka, J. N., et al. Cardiorespiratory fitness and adiposity as mortality predictors in older adults. *JAMA* 298, no. 21 (December 5, 2007): 2507–16.

index

Underscored page references indicate sidebars. **Boldface** references indicate photographs and illustrations.

F

Falls, preventing, 22, 23, 30
Family member, as workout
  buddy, 62
Fat, body
  muscle tone replacing, 21–22
  yoga reducing, 76
Fat Blast walks, 31, 32, 80, 85, 106
Fat burning, factors increasing
  cardio exercise, xviii–xix
  sleep, 41, 55
  weight training, 17, 20
Fatigue
  chronic, 23
  from using weights, 25
Fats, dietary, types of, 207. *see also*
  MUFAs; Saturated fats
Fidgeting, calorie burning from,
  164
Fight-or-flight response, 46, 47,
  178
Fish
  on Flat Belly Diet! shopping
    list, 231
  as lean protein, 225
Fitness community, joining, 62
Flat Belly Diet!
  changing thoughts about
    eating, xv
  diseases prevented by, 207
  effectiveness of, viii
  Flat Belly Yoga! Workout
    combined with, xiii, 74,
    205, 206, 212, 235, 240,
    242–43, 249
  flexibility of, 233–35
  4-Day Anti-Bloat Jump Start
    in (*see* 4-Day Anti-Bloat
    Jump Start)
  4-Week Meal Plan in (*see*
    4-Week Meal Plan)
  guidelines for following,
    209–11
  MUFAs in, xii, 208 (*see also*
    MUFAs)
  reasons for success with, 211–12
  rules for following, 208–9
  shopping list for, 228–32
  success stories about, 236–37,
    242–43
Flat Belly Diet!, 206, 209, 213,
  220, 221, 224, 226, 233

Flat Belly Diet! Cookbook, 209, 221
Flat Belly Diet! Pocket Guide,
  209, 221, 226, 232
Flat Belly for Life
  benefits of following, 244–47
  deciding to follow, 240–41
  inspiration for, 250
  rules for, 247–50
Flat Belly Yoga!
  options after reading, 239–41
  purpose and goals of, vii, ix,
    xii–xiii, xiv, xix, 12, 13,
    60
  reason for interest in, xi, xii,
    76, 187
flatbellyyoga.com, 250
Flat Belly Yoga! Journal. *See also*
  Journaling
  for Core+ Yoga routine, 118
  for Flat Belly for Life, 250
  for 4-Day Jump Start, 84,
    184–85, 186
  for 4-Week Workout, 187–201
  how to keep, 182–83, 201
  purpose of, 177, 181, 202–3
    changing negative
      thoughts, 41
    finding best time for
      workouts, 54, 79
    finding time for exercise,
      168, 181–82
    identifying imbalances in
      body, 66
    identifying stressors, 46
    recording excuses for
      inactivity, 80
    tracking Heart Walks, 80
Flat Belly Yoga! program. *See*
  also Flat Belly Yoga!
  Workout; Yoga
  continuing, after 4-week
    program, 243 (*see also*
    Flat Belly for Life)
  indulgences and, 233
  for losing belly fat, vii, xii, xiii,
    21, 55, 76, 206
  recording weight and
    measurements before
    starting, 69, 69
  results after completing, 240,
    241
  success stories about (*see*
    Success stories)

Flat Belly Yoga! Workout. *See*
  also Flat Belly Yoga!
  program; Yoga
  benefits of, 39, 50–51, 76
  best time to do, 79
  breathing technique for, 3
  changing mindset for, xv
  components of, ix, xvii, 13, 17
    (*see also* Flat Belly Yoga!
    Workout; 4-Day Flat
    Belly Yoga! Jump Start;
    4-Week Workout; Heart
    Walks)
  Flat Belly Diet! combined
    with, xiii, 74, 205, 206,
    212, 235, 240, 242–43,
    249
  making time for, 75–76
  music for, 41, 42–43, 44–45
  poses in, 6–11 (*see also* Yoga
    for Your Core Routine;
    *specific Core+ Yoga
    routines*)
  progressions in, 60
  reason for doing, 251
  rules for, 59
    finding workout buddy,
      61–63
    having fun, 61–63
    making realistic plans, 61
    starting small, 60
  starting tips for, xiii–xv, 80
Flaxseed oil, 222
Flexibility, yoga improving, 2
Food colorings, artificial,
  avoiding, 210
Forward Bend, Standing, **122**,
  132, **132**, **148**
4-Day Anti-Bloat Jump Start
  menus for, 213, 216–19
  principles of
    avoiding banned foods, 215,
      215
    drinking Sassy Water, 214
    eating four 300-calorie
      meals per day, 214
    eating slowly, 214–15
    following 4-day meal plan,
      213
  purpose of, 212
  results from, 220
  workout combined with, 74,
    249

Memory
   strength training improving, 23–24
   stress hormones impairing, 45
Memory loss, walking preventing, 31
Menopause, 21, 22, 245
Menus
   for 4-Day Anti-Bloat Jump Start, 213, 216–19
   for 4-Week Meal Plan, 226
Metabolism boosters
   interval exercise, 31
   meal frequency, 209
   weight training, 17, 18, 19, 104
Mind-Belly Connection, 45–54, 180, 192
Mini-lifts. *See* Warrior 2 with Mini-Lifts
Monounsaturated fatty acids. *See* MUFAs
Mood boosters
   exercise, 30, 45, 46, 244–45
   yoga boosting, 2, 53
Motivation. *See also* Mat Motivations
   behind goals, xiv
   journaling for, 182, 202
   positive attitude for, 41
   stress preventing, 45
   for walking, 63, 80
   for workouts, 84, 244
      belonging to fitness community, 62
      Core Confidences for, 187–201
      lack of, 63
      writing about, 181
MUFAs
   categories of
      avocados, 208, 211, 221, 224
      dark chocolate, 208, 211, 221, 224
      nuts and seeds, 208, 211, 221, 222–23
      oils, 208, 211, 221, 222
      olives, 208, 211, 221, 224
   in every meal, 209
   health benefits of, 207
   for losing visceral fat, xii
   meal building and, 211–12, 220, 221, **221**
   swapping, 233–34, 237

Muscle loss, with aging, xviii, 20, 21, 245
Muscle mass
   benefits of, 17, 19, 20, 21–22
   Flat Belly Yoga! for building, xii, xviii, 11, 18, 104, 108
   process of building, 20, 22
Muscles, core. *See* Core muscles
Muscular strength, yoga improving, 2
Music
   for Flat Belly Yoga! workouts, 41, 42–43, 44–45, 189, 196
   for Heart Walks, 44, 63, 84, 99, 191, 196
   safety while listening to, 44, 67
   for Yoga for Your Core, 84, 99

N

Neely, Paul, success story of, 174–75, **174**, **175**
Negative emotions, from working out, 178–79
Negative self-talk loop, 179
Negative thoughts
   eliminating, 183, 187, 196
   journaling about, 179
   managing, 41
Nuts
   buying, 222
   in Flat Belly Diet!, 208, 210, 211, 221, 222–23
   storing, 222
   toasting, 223
   uses for, 222–23

O

Obesity
   from irregular eating patterns, 168
   subcutaneous fat with, xii
Oils, in Flat Belly Diet!, 208, 211, 221, 222
Olive oil, in Flat Belly Diet!, 210, 222
Olives, in Flat Belly Diet!, 208, 211, 221, 224

Omega-3 fats, in fish, 225
Optimism
   exercise creating, 50
   stress prevention from, 41
Organic foods
   fruits and vegetables, 227
   meats, 225
Osteoporosis, 22, 225
Overhead lifts. *See* Warrior 1 with Overhead Lifts
Overweight, subcutaneous fat with, xii

P

Pain. *See also* Injuries
   absent from Core+ workouts, 19
   back, 5, 15, 26
   exercise-related, endorphins reducing, 63
   from yoga, avoiding, 64
   yoga relieving, 26, 54
Parasympathetic nervous system
   for relaxation, 53
   stress and, 47
Peanut butter, 223
Peanut oil, 222
Peanuts, 223
Pecans, 223
   Baby Green Pocket, 226
Phone conversations
   during walks, 63, 169, 169
   yoga poses during, 172
Physical inactivity, statistics on, 241
Pineapple Smoothie, 217, 219
Pine nuts, 223
   Hummus Dip, 226
Pistachios, 223
Plank Pose
   in Core+ Flow, 134, **134**
   core strength for holding, 14
   description of, 8
   extending hold in, 172
Plateaus, fitness, 41
Play It Safe tips
   avoiding food rewards, 235
   for avoiding injury, 2
   doctor approval for exercise, 13

Weight training
    benefits of, 17–18, 19–25
    in Core+ workouts, xviii, 13, 17
    starting tips for, 18–19
    in yoga-hybrid workout, 18
Whole grains, in Flat Belly Diet!
        meals, 227
Williams, Nicole, 26
    success story of, 36–37, **36, 37**
Williams, Robert, 36
    success story of, 26–27, **26, 27**
Windshield Wiper
    how to do, 96, **96**
    in Yoga for Your Core Routine,
        86
Women
    bone loss in, 22, 30, 225
    heart disease in, 77
    menopause and, 21, 22, 245
    muscle and, 19, 21–22
    self-care and, 75
    self-criticism by, 40–41
Workout buddies, 35, 35, 61–63,
        189
Workouts. *See also* Flat Belly
        Yoga! Workout; *specific*
        Core+ Yoga workouts
    benefits of, xv–xvi, 103
    commitment to, xiii, xiv, xv,
        76, 107, 183, 246
    craving for, xvi
    finding time for (*see* Time for
        workouts)
    hybrid, viii–ix, xviii, 18, 83
    increasing enjoyment of, 189
    motivation for, 84, 244
        belonging to fitness
            community, 62

Core Confidences
    providing, 187–201
    lack of, 63
    positive self-talk about,
        xvi–xvii
    writing about, 181 (*see also*
        Flat Belly Yoga! Journal)
Writing, in journal. *See* Flat Belly
        Yoga! Journal;
        Journaling

Y

YAS Fitness Center, viii, ix, 13,
        62, 83, 248
Yoga. *See also* Flat Belly Yoga!
        program; Flat Belly Yoga
        Workout!
    breathing in, 3, 7, 66, 84
    classes, 12
    clothing for, 65
    emotional releases from,
        179
    as habit, 75–76
    health benefits of, xvii, 2, 76
        sleep improvement, 54
        stress relief, 2, 3, 45, 53
    hybrid forms of, viii–ix, 18, 83
    mainstream acceptance of,
        1–2
    preventing injuries from, 2, 18,
        64, 74, 172, 202
    rules for
        finding right location, 64
        focusing on breath, 66
        maintaining body
            awareness, 65–66

    observing limits, 64
    warming up, 64–65
    styles of, 12–13
    weights combined with, 24
Yoga for Athletes, 13
Yoga for Your Core Routine
    form check for, 84
    in 4-Day Jump Start, xvii, 64,
        73
    goal of, 11
    incorporated in 4-Week
        Workout, 79
    for injury prevention, 2
    location and equipment for, 86
    music for, 84, 99
    poses in
        Bridge with a Lift, **86**, 97,
            97
        Chair Pose, **86**, 91, **91**
        Corpse, **87**, 98, **98**
        Easy Spinal Twist, **87**, 89,
            89
        Hero Pose with a Lift, **87**,
            93, **93**
        Rock Up to Standing, **87**,
            90, **90**
        Seated Tree-Up and Over,
            87, 94–95, **94–95**
        Warm-Up/Breath Work,
            86, 88, **88**
        Warrior 1, **86**, 92, **92**
        Windshield Wiper, **86**, 96,
            96
    stress relief from, 51
    weights excluded from, 18
Yoga-with-weights workouts, ix,
        xvii, 13, 24, 161. *See also*
        4-Week Workout